Published by: 3 Bar Press, A Division and Imprint of Marketing for Solos®
6767 South Spruce Street, Suite #205, Centennial, Colorado, 80112.

First Edition
ISBN-10: 0-9769962-1-9
ISBN-13: 978-0-9769962-1-7

Printed in the United States of America.
10 9 8 7 6 5 4 3 2 1

What Others Say About This Book

"I highly recommend this book—it's easy to understand and is an inspiring read. These patients' stories offer evidence that better health is possible for those who are suffering from thyroid symptoms."

— **Julie Brown,** DC, DACNB
Southern California Brain Center
Los Alamitos, California
www.SoCalBrainCenter.com

"Thyroid problems are often complex. For healing to happen, a practitioner must dig deep to understand each patient's condition. This book is filled with stories that will help guide patients as they seek a practitioner who understands how to manage the root cause of their health conditions."

— **A. Elliot Hirshorn, III,** DC, DACNB, DPSc
New Life Functional Neurology & Endocrinology
Simpsonville, South Carolina
www.RenewingFunction.com

"As a practitioner who also helps patients with thyroid problems, it's refreshing to read a book that is not overly complicated or full of medical jargon. This book is a great resource for readers who want to understand thyroid dysfunction. I recommend this book to anyone who needs help improving his or her thyroid health."

— **Randy Hansbrough,** DC, DACAN, FIACN, CFMP
Hansbrough Functional Neurology
Stuart, Florida
www.HCFN.org

"Fantastic! Dr. Redd's book is full of success stories that will help readers gain insight into thyroid health. I highly recommend it."

— **Russell J. Kort,** DC
Kort Chiropractic and Rehab
Sherwood, Oregon
www.KortChiropractic.com

"A wonderful book that spells out the steps to take when searching for thyroid health. No one should ever give up in the search for health, healing and wellness."

— **Jeremy Schmoe,** DC, DACNB, FACFN
Minnesota Functional Neurology and Chiropractic
Minneapolis, Minnesota
www.MinnesotaFunctionalNeurology.com

"Dr. Redd has put together a no-nonsense approach to thyroid dysfunction that will help put patients on the path to improved health. This book spells out the truth about low thyroid in a way that is easy to understand and easy to apply."

— **John Rees,** DC, CFMP
Functional Chiropractic
Milton, Delaware
www.FunctionalWellnessDelmarva.com

"This book is simple and easy to understand. It has a wealth of inspiring stories. It is a great education on thyroid health and explains why so many patients with thyroid problems go undiagnosed or misdiagnosed and mismanaged. Well done, Dr. Redd."

— **Robin Schaefer,** DC, LAc
Aurora Wellness Center
Aurora, Oregon
www.Aurora-Wellness.com

Table of Contents

. . . .

. . . .

Acknowledgements

First and foremost, none of these success stories would be possible without the direction and methods organized by Datis Kharrazian, DHSc, DC, MS. I thank him and his team for empowering me with the necessary tools to provide thorough diagnoses and effective condition management to patients who suffer from thyroid conditions. Dr. Kharrazian and his team have helped me become the doctor I am today.

Next, I thank the doctors of RedRiver Health and Wellness Center, who work fervently to provide our patients with the best quality of care: Brinton Andersen, DC, DABFM; Josh Conzo, DC, CFMP; Brooke Conzo, DC, CFMP; Samuel Gage, DC, MS, DABFM, DAAIM; Paul Stadler, DC; and Jeremy Swindlehurst, DC.

I extend my sincere gratitude to the courageous patients who have shared their stories on the following pages; without their contributions, this book would not have been possible.

Additionally, I thank each and every patient who has put his or her trust in RedRiver Health and Wellness Center over the years—you are the reason we do what we do.

To my regional manager, Julyn Watkins, I extend special thanks for being an integral part of RedRiver Health and Wellness Center, for helping compile and edit the contents of this book, and for consistently making my life easier.

I thank Rebecca Hart for contributing her writing and editing talents to this project.

I express my appreciation to the many people and organizations that provided support, feedback, and direction throughout the publishing process of this book, including Marketing for Solos®.

Most importantly, I thank my beautiful wife, Brittany. She has been my inspiration and motivation for continuing to improve my knowledge, which allows me to move forward in my career. Her compassion and love enable me to spend countless hours doing what I am passionate about—helping others.

Foreword

By Dr. Shane Steadman

In my experience as a chiropractic neurologist and functional medicine practitioner, I have had the privilege of helping many patients with thyroid disorders reclaim their lives. Thyroid conditions, which are often overlooked, can be quite frustrating for patients, especially for those who have been suffering for years. Unfortunately, there is no "magic pill" or "quick fix" for thyroid dysfunction. Whether patients are experiencing headaches, chronic fatigue, insomnia, GI disorders, or other debilitating symptoms, I use the fundamental principles of functional medicine to teach patients about their thyroid conditions and help them mange their health.

Dr. Joshua Redd shares my passion for helping individuals with chronic health conditions. He has received training from some of the leading functional medicine practitioners in the country, including Dr. Datis Kharrazian. Dr. Redd's knowledge, experience, and compassion allow him to help patients achieve long-term wellness. He runs a reputable practice with a number of locations in the United States, and he and his team of health practitioners have helped countless patients reclaim their health.

The Truth About Low Thyroid sheds light on the primary cause of thyroid dysfunction, and offers insight and direction to those experiencing unexplained or unresolved symptoms. This book shows readers that they're not suffering alone—there are so many people out there who are experiencing debilitating symptoms related to thyroid disorders.

If you or loved ones have symptoms that are affecting your quality of life, please read these stories. Let this book inspire you to seek out help, because better health is possible if you don't give up.

Shane Steadman, DC, DACNB, DCBCN, DCCN, FAAIM, FACFN, CNS
Board Certified Chiropractic Neurologist
Owner of Integrated Health Systems, Denver, CO
Owner of Integrated Brain Systems, Denver, CO

Introduction

What you're about to read are the personal stories of several of my patients in their own words. Of course, it's hard to share these stories without sounding biased about our clinic and the work we do with our patients. That is certainly not my intention in writing this book. My intention is to help you get to the truth about low thyroid.

What you will learn from, and likely relate to, are the heartfelt stories of real people who may have experienced some of the same health struggles that you have. These men and women grew more and more frustrated as their health spiraled downward, and many of them felt so hopeless that they were at the end of their ropes. Through perseverance and determination, these individuals continued to search until they found the tools necessary to finally get their health back on track.

My goal is to increase awareness about the help available to you or your loved ones who are struggling with similar health problems. Throughout this book, I have included Redd Flags of information and commentary. These Redd Flags are designed to enhance your understanding of the circumstances and medical factors involved in each patient's story. I want you to be inspired and empowered to seek help for your health concerns, and I want you to find the courage to regain hope.

Joshua Redd, DC, MS, DABFM, DAAIM
Chiropractic Physician
Owner & Founder of RedRiver Health and Wellness Center

CHAPTER 1

Why This Book?

When I first decided to write about low thyroid, I planned to write a comprehensive book about the leading cause of low thyroid in America. (I explain what that cause is in Chapter 2.) I was going to include an in-depth look into immunological, biological, and biochemical research, and I planned to explain the various reasons so many people continue to suffer with low thyroid symptoms despite being on thyroid medication.

There are several books available that address thyroid disorders from a medical standpoint, and many of these books are full of valuable information. One such book, which I highly recommend, is *Why Do I Still Have Thyroid Symptoms When My Lab Tests are Normal: a Revolutionary Breakthrough in Understanding Hashimoto's Disease and Hypothyroidism* by Datis Kharrazian, DHSc, DC, MS.

Once I sat down to begin writing, I realized I wanted to approach this book differently. I wanted my book to be about something more than research and data. I wanted to focus on something we hear in our offices every day: the stories of patients suffering from low thyroid symptoms. These patients often come in to our offices feeling so unwell that they can't imagine living healthy, happy lives. Many patients arrive in tears and without adequate words to describe how they feel and what they have experienced.

There are so many people out there who have lost all hope—they have seen practitioner after practitioner, but haven't been able to feel better, and they have done countless hours of research without finding the answers they desperately need. Fortunately, wellness may very well be within their reach.

For this reason, I wanted to write a book about real people who never give up and never give in. A book that offers guidance to those who dream of feeling better. A book about faith and healing for those suffering with low thyroid symptoms. A book about the truth—the truth about low thyroid. The truth is, there is hope; there is help for those who continue to suffer from low thyroid symptoms.

If you or your loved ones are suffering with low thyroid symptoms, this book will encourage you to keep going and guide you to the help you are seeking. Do not give up. Do not give in. Do not lose hope.

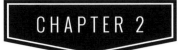

CHAPTER 2

The Truth About Low Thyroid

The truth about low thyroid is that low thyroid is often caused by an autoimmune condition or an imbalance somewhere else in the body.[2,4]

If you are like many people, you have gone to a healthcare professional with common low thyroid symptoms such as extreme fatigue, the need for excessive amounts of sleep in order to function, weight gain (even when eating healthy and exercising regularly), thin or brittle hair, hair loss (especially the outside portion of the eyebrows), low libido, brain fog or memory problems, insomnia, depression, anxiety, trouble regulating body temperature, headaches, and/or chronic digestive problems.[3,4,5]

The healthcare provider ran TSH markers—maybe even a T3 and T4—to see how your thyroid was working. When your results came back, you may have been told that your lab tests and blood work were

Thyroid
A butterfly-shaped gland at the front of the neck that regulates body functions, including metabolism.[1]

Autoimmune Condition
A condition where the body's immune system attacks itself.[2]

TSH
Thyroid stimulating hormone; a TSH test measures the amount of thyroid stimulating hormone in the blood.[3]

Hashimoto's Disease
Autoimmune disease of the thyroid.[1]

"normal." You were probably not made aware of any other options available to address your specific symptoms. If your levels were not in the "normal" range, you may have been put on a thyroid medication, but many of the symptoms did not go away or may have become more severe.

So how can it be that so many people still suffer from low thyroid symptoms even when they are on medications or under the care of a healthcare professional? It is because many low thyroid patients also suffer from an autoimmune condition called Hashimoto's disease.[4,5] In cases of Hashimoto's disease, medications typically do not alleviate thyroid symptoms because they do not address the root cause of the condition.

In Fact, Hashimoto's Disease Is the #1 Cause of Low Thyroid in America

Hashimoto's disease is an autoimmune condition—where the body's immune system attacks healthy tissues—that destroys thyroid tissue. When the immune system attacks the thyroid for an extended period of time, the thyroid loses its ability to function properly. If the thyroid doesn't function properly, it can no longer produce the life-sustaining thyroid hormones the body needs.[4] For those with Hashimoto's disease, the thyroid is not the culprit; it is just the victim of a much bigger problem.

Because the thyroid itself is not the problem in these cases, you'll hear of patients going from one healthcare provider to another, having test after test, and taking medication after medication, even as their quality of life continues to decline.

This is the unfortunate story we often hear from those seeking help from RedRiver Health and Wellness Center, and this is what happened to the patients you will read about in this book. These patients suffered from Hashimoto's disease, not simply low thyroid.

The truth about low thyroid is that if you are on thyroid medication and still have symptoms, if you have had your TSH levels tested and your healthcare provider says they are "normal" but you still have symptoms, or if you continually suffer from low thyroid without relief, then the odds are that you may have Hashimoto's disease.[6(p.42)]

Having a Mechanistic Approach Rather Than a Condition or Symptom Approach

As a chiropractic physician who uses functional medicine techniques, I have devoted my professional career to helping patients who suffer from challenging conditions. I understand that we can't simply minimize symptoms and expect to get long-term results; instead, my team and I dig much deeper to determine the root cause of each patient's health problems. We take into consideration the underlying physiological mechanisms causing each patient's condition or symptoms, and we examine physiological imbalances that may have been previously overlooked.

When we see a patient who is suffering from low thyroid and has symptoms that aren't improving with traditional care, we, as healthcare providers, should ask ourselves, "What is the underlying mechanism that is causing this problem?"

Once we identify that mechanism to be Hashimoto's disease, we must then ask, "What are the imbalances that are causing this patient's immune system to become hyperactive and attack the thyroid?" Answering this question requires detailed testing and analysis to pinpoint the specific factors causing the patient's disease to flare up and manifest symptoms.

If a healthcare practitioner does not find out what is causing the patient's Hashimoto's to attack the thyroid, it is difficult to facilitate relief. Again, this is why we see so many patients who have normal TSH levels but still feel terrible. In many cases, they are getting worse and worse because their immune systems are raging uncontrollably through their bodies, attacking otherwise healthy tissues. The best way to describe Hashimoto's symptoms is like a fire alarm going off to warn us of a house fire; medications may turn off the alarm temporarily, but they don't extinguish the fire that is destroying the house.

It is important to find a healthcare provider who will follow the four-step process listed below; this allows the practitioner to discover the root cause of the patient's symptoms and efficiently manage the condition:

1. Order comprehensive lab tests, including tests for Hashimoto's disease. To check for Hashimoto's, thyroid peroxidase antibody (TPO) and antithyroglobulin antibody tests must be ordered.[9(p.58)] If these tests are positive for Hashimoto's disease, additional lab work should be ordered to identify the triggers that flare up the patient's disease.
2. Analyze the test results using functional ranges.
3. Customize a care plan for the patient based on his or her specific needs with the goal of reducing inflammation to calm the autoimmune response.
4. Teach and educate the patient about Hashimoto's disease— what it does and how it impacts the thyroid, body function, and overall health—to empower the patient to be actively involved in his or her own health.

Hashimoto's disease is a complex autoimmune condition. There is much work that goes into evaluating the way the disease affects each individual patient, and into managing the disease itself. It is rarely found to be an isolated condition. A person may have several imbalances occurring all at once, and each one must be addressed. These imbalances can range from liver dysfunction, hormonal imbalances, intestinal problems, genetic polymorphisms, inflammation, mitochondrial dysfunction, oxidative stress, and neuroendocrine immune imbalances to factors as seemingly simple as food sensitivities, emotional stressors, and environmental reactions.

The inherent complexity of concurrent imbalances is the reason patients on symptom-based medications may feel little to no improvement; in these cases, the main mechanism—Hashimoto's—and the underlying imbalances that are feeding off each other are being completely overlooked.

The truth about low thyroid is that you may have Hashimoto's disease, and Hashimoto's may be the cause of your symptoms.

What if You Truly Have a Permanent Low Thyroid?

Every cell in your body has a thyroid hormone receptor site, and thyroid hormone is crucial for the optimal function of your entire body.[1] *If your healthcare provider has diagnosed you with a permanent low thyroid, it is important that you do not discontinue your medication or hormone replacement therapy without consulting the prescribing medical professional.* In cases where Hashimoto's has damaged the thyroid, the gland can no longer produce the life-sustaining hormones the body needs and is dependent upon the prescribed thyroid hormone.

There are many cases where thyroid hormone medications are necessary, and those patients who have a permanent low thyroid must be managed with medication. Even in these cases, it is important to remember that thyroid medication does nothing to address the autoimmune disease itself, and does not address any other factors that have caused the thyroid problem. So, if a healthcare professional is simply prescribing a thyroid hormone while neglecting the root cause of the low thyroid, the patient may continue to get worse.

For patients suffering with low thyroid caused by Hashimoto's disease, some of the biggest improvements happen when we co-manage their care with a prescribing health professional. For some of the patients whose stories you will read, thyroid medication began to work much more effectively once we addressed the chaotic mess of imbalances and symptoms caused by Hashimoto's. Once the autoimmunity is calmed, the body has the ability to metabolize thyroid hormone much more efficiently.

There Is Hope

Remember, there is hope. There is help. There is healing. If you're still experiencing low thyroid symptoms while taking medication, there is a good chance you have an underlying condition that is not being addressed.

We see patients every day who have heard from a healthcare provider, "Take this pill—there's nothing more to do." When this happens, the patient leaves that office without answers and often feels frustrated and hopeless. Patients who experience this generally don't realize they are likely to have Hashimoto's disease; they don't realize that, if their low thyroid is caused by an autoimmune condition, there are many things that can be done to help them improve. These improvements are sometimes dramatic. The most important things to remember are:

If you have been diagnosed with low thyroid, ask your healthcare provider to test you for Hashimoto's disease.

If you are diagnosed with Hashimoto's disease, it is imperative that your healthcare provider appropriately addresses your condition. Unmanaged autoimmunity predisposes you to additional autoimmune diseases.[7]

If you are suffering from low thyroid and/or Hashimoto's disease, working with the right healthcare provider is crucial. If you are able to find a medical professional who can provide you with honest, informed answers and appropriate management strategies, it is possible to achieve a better quality of life and a drastically improved health outcome. A functional medicine or personalized lifestyle medicine provider who focuses on identifying and addressing the root cause of your condition (instead of just your symptoms) may be the answer.

The truth is, Hashimoto's disease is the leading cause of low thyroid in America.[5] The truth is, there is a different way—a way of hope and healing and answers. No matter which healthcare provider you choose to work with, make sure you find the truth. Your truth.

Common Symptoms of Hashimoto's Disease and Low Thyroid

SYMPTOM	HASHIMOTO'S	LOW THYROID
Fatigue	✔	✔
Brain Fog	✔	✔
Weight Gain	✔	✔
Hair Loss	✔	✔
Headaches	✔	✔
Feeling Cold	✔	✔
Constipation	✔	✔
Dry Skin	✔	✔
Depression	✔	✔
Low Libido	✔	✔
Abnormal Menstruation	✔	✔
Joint Pain	✔	
Heart Palpitations	✔	
Hoarse Voice	✔	
Volatile Weight Change	✔	
Poor Sleep Patterns	✔	
Fullness in Throat	✔	
Enlarged Thyroid Gland	✔	

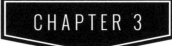

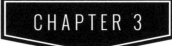

It's Never Too Late in Life to Feel Healthy

Linda's Story

Retired math tutor, Linda, is an inspiring example of one very important truth about low thyroid conditions: it's never too late to feel healthy! For more than 60 years, Linda struggled with debilitating health problems related to food and dieting. She was physically and spiritually weakened to a point from which she doubted she could ever recover.

Today, Linda is grateful she never gave up her search for wellness, even when it seemed like there was nothing left to do. Now, at the age of 72, Linda's health has been completely transformed. Her energy and enthusiasm belie her age, and she exudes a zest for life.

◇◇◇◇◇◇◇◇◇◇◇◇◇◇◇◇◇◇◇◇◇◇◇◇

"Over and over I was told the same thing: 'Your thyroid is fine. You shouldn't be putting on all this weight. Stop eating so much, and get some exercise.' When I was finally put on thyroid replacement, they increased my dosage every time I started to feel worse. It didn't do any good."

◇◇◇◇◇◇◇◇◇◇◇◇◇◇◇◇◇◇◇◇◇◇◇◇

Growing up, my family life was centered on food. My mother made sure we had desserts all the time. If we didn't have cookies in the cupboard, she made frosting and put it between graham crackers to hand out as treats. That was the way she showed us love—through food.

Looking back to my earliest memories, I can see the seeds of my lifetime struggle with dieting and food. I remember being at a doctor's office at the age of four. He pointed his finger at me and said, "You're so fat, you'll never be able to eat Jell-O or avocados again!" I was just a naughty little fat girl to him. That's when it all began.

My unhealthy eating habits started early, and I developed a skewed attitude toward food. Combined with what was likely a metabolic problem, I was in bad straights as a kid.

Although I was overweight as a child, I did lose the weight once I hit puberty and became active in cheerleading and musicals. Looking back at photos of my high school and college years, I remember struggling to lose weight. I recognize now that my weight was perfectly normal, but at the time I was constantly thinking, "I have to lose weight." And what happened as a result? I dieted and starved myself into obesity. I had metabolic problems, and I messed my body up even more with one starvation diet after another.

I was 22 years old when I had my first child—the first of six babies— and I started packing on weight. I gained more than 200 pounds over the next 40 years, and my health plummeted. Adrenal fatigue knocked me out, and I was constantly stressed and exhausted. I was also pre-diabetic.

My healthcare provider's solution was to prescribe an antidepressant to help with my anxiety and fatigue. I suppose the pills "worked" in that I became numb to everything, but I knew it wasn't natural to feel that way. I didn't like it. I decided I'd rather deal with depression and low energy than cover up what was really happening.

I tried to walk or run, which was what I'd always done to help relieve stress, but I started having terrible pain in my knees. I became more and more isolated as my weight kept climbing; I couldn't handle being in crowds. I was overwhelmed just getting out of bed in the morning—it was something I had to force myself to do.

I knew something was drastically wrong. I went from one doctor to another and had my thyroid tested again and again. Over and over I was told the same thing: "Your thyroid is fine. You shouldn't be putting on all this weight. Stop eating so much, and get some exercise." When I was finally put on thyroid replacement, they increased my dosage every time I started to feel worse. It didn't do any good.

Again and again I was told, "There's no reason for you to be feeling as bad as you do. It's all in your head." It's difficult to explain the impact of being told over and over that you're basically imagining things. I was hanging on to my life with my fingernails and felt just like I had as a four-year-old kid—fat. This time, instead of "naughty," I felt crazy.

My life was a roller coaster ride as I tried one starvation diet after another. I tried high fat and low fat, high carbs and low carbs—I swear, there isn't a diet plan on earth I haven't abused my body with. I even entered a hospital program where I consumed nothing but protein shakes for four and a half months. I had not one crumb of food. Can you imagine? It's tough to think

Redd Flag

If you've tried diet after diet and you're still gaining weight, a metabolic imbalance may be the cause. One possibility is that you have an autoimmune low thyroid condition that has shut down the hormone-sensitive lipase enzyme (HSL) that breaks down fat in the body.[8]

It's also common for autoimmune low thyroid patients to experience insulin resistance.[9] The patient eats a meal, which turns into glucose. This glucose should enter into the body's cells to be used for energy, but the glucose can't enter the cells efficiently because of the insulin resistance, so the body turns it into fat.[10]

This is a double-edged sword for patients trying to lose weight. No matter how much they exercise or how little they eat, they still gain weight. Here are some things to look for if this sounds like you:

1. Autoimmune Low Thyroid
2. Insulin Resistance
3. PCOS – Polycystic Ovarian Syndrome
4. Increased testosterone in females and increased estrogen in males
5. Poor gut microbiota

about the horrible example I set for my kids.

Still, I refused to give up my search for better health because I so badly wanted to enjoy some kind of quality of life. I went round and round with various hormone replacement therapies, dosages, and a whole slew of antidepressants—but it was all like a big, sad joke. The longer things went on, the worse I felt.

I developed terrible insomnia, which only made my physical exhaustion worse. I was so intolerant of cold that I always wore a sweater. The aches and pains in my knees spread to all my muscles and joints. My memory started to fade. I had brain fog so bad, I couldn't remember people's names, and I forgot words for common things and situations.

When menopause hit and the children married and left home, we moved south to a warmer part of Utah. I was barely getting through the days trying to do the bare minimum around the house—preparing meals and doing some housework. I couldn't do much because pain ruled my body. It's hard to look back at those years. I feel bad. There's so much I missed out on. It was all I could do to get through a simple activity like washing dishes, let alone get to family outings or participate in social activities.

I'm not exaggerating when I say I've struggled through a lifetime of obsession with food and dieting and trying to find "the answer." I have felt so lousy and lived with so much shame and guilt. I've studied nutrition and health for decades, and I have more books on these topics than most libraries. When you feel as bad as I have, the search for answers becomes that serious and that deep—it can become an obsession.

I've met many people with severe weight and health problems over the years. I know it's common for them to feel like giving up, and I don't blame them. When healthcare professionals keep telling you there's nothing wrong and there's nothing they can do to help, something else has to keep you going. That drive for me was a spiritual one. I held on to the belief that I could become healthy. I clung to the belief that out of my weakness, something good would come. I thought someday, maybe

I could be an instrument to help other people. I knew that what I'd physically suffered with all my life was my weakness. I had faith that if I could just find the right approach or combination of approaches, that weakness could become a strength. I hung onto that belief, and I kept going.

In November of 2011, my health had deteriorated to the point where I was approaching death's door. Sometimes I had to be in a wheelchair. The pain of just getting out of bed in the morning was overwhelming. I was emotionally exhausted from battling what went into my mouth and what didn't. It felt like life was no longer worth waking up for; I was closer than I'd ever been to giving up.

At that point, I felt like I had nothing left to lose. I was in excruciating pain that tore at my joints, knees and muscles. It felt like the pain was attacking my bones. I'd failed to find a solution. It felt like there was nothing more I could do, but my prayers, faith, and scripture study blessed me with this miraculous experience:

One night, I was tossing and turning in bed as usual, suffering with pain and insomnia. I felt the need to get myself out of bed and turn on the TV. It wasn't easy; I had to literally drag myself over to a chair by the TV.

I started flipping through shows I had recorded and landed on one I'd never seen. I knew I didn't record it, but I decided to watch it anyway. It turned out to be a healthcare advisor interviewing one of his patients on a morning show. As I listened to this patient, I realized she was telling my story. She could have

> ## Redd Flag
> Some of our patients have found that relying on a higher power has helped in their healing process. If you have an interest or inclination toward exploring spirituality in general or specific ways, it's possible doing so may be of assistance in your outcome, too.[11]

been talking about my life—our experiences were that similar. I wrote down the name of this practitioner, and called his office the very next morning.

The office turned out to be about a four-hour drive from where I lived, but I knew I had to talk to this healthcare professional. I scheduled a consultation and sent my blood work to the office so he would have the results when it came time for my appointment.

The practitioner called me for my consultation, and hearing him speak was like a confirmation that I was finally on the right path. He sounded energetic, upbeat, positive and confident. Trust and hope washed over my body from the top of my head to my toes. It was an incredible experience.

He told me I had Hashimoto's disease, and that my blood tests revealed multiple imbalances. I needed a lot of help, but I was three hundred miles away and I couldn't even walk. It was excruciatingly painful, awkward, and awful for me to get in the car, never mind travel that far. I knew the colder temperatures at the office location would aggravate my whole body, but I was determined to get there.

On the day of my appointment, I could barely hobble into the office. That first office appointment was comforting, and gave me so much hope. I'd seen dozens of health professionals over the years; never had I met one who was so friendly, energetic, and, most importantly, nonjudgmental.

He was respectful and helped me get out of my chair to be weighed. I joked that his scale probably didn't go up high enough, since my weight was so out of control, but he wasn't surprised at what I weighed. There were no disapproving looks; there was no finger wagging. To him, my weight was simply the result of my body's poor condition. He was confident my weight was something that could be addressed as I healed. It felt like coming home!

I'm grateful every day that I found him. The funny thing is, when I went back to look at that interview again—the recording I watched in the middle of the night—it was nowhere to be found.

I started my new healthcare plan right away. It's unreal, but I started feeling better within two weeks. I felt like I'd been plugged into an energy outlet; all of a sudden I was awake! Every day, I felt myself coming out of the deep, dark abyss I'd lived in for decades. My body felt like it did a complete turnaround.

I knew about calories in and calories out, and even that the quality of the calories makes a difference, but I learned that there was so much more to it. My immune system was reacting to a bunch of foods I considered healthy, and calorie counts and quality didn't matter as long as I was taking in those inflammatory foods. No wonder I had been feeling worse and worse! My body hadn't been absorbing nutrients. I had craved sugars and starches because I literally wasn't getting the energy necessary to fuel my body. I had no way of knowing this before meeting my new healthcare practitioner, because no other medical professional had ever bothered to look.

All it really took for me to start to heal and feel well was finally discovering my body's truth. My healthcare advisor helped me find that truth, and my body naturally responded.

My care lasted nearly a year because my body was in such an unhealthy state. But here it is, almost three years since I started, and I'm able to take care of myself. I've learned so much about what my body needs, and why, that I can manage my own health. My practitioner never said, "Just do what I say." Instead, he taught me the truth about my own body!

Everything has changed for the better. I've released 85 pounds. My pain has diminished, and I sleep better. I can handle stress, and my gastrointestinal problems have been addressed so I'm able to absorb nutrients when I eat. For the first time in my life, I can tell when I'm full and when I'm still hungry. Before, I had no idea. I could eat and eat and eat, and never feel satisfied. Now, my body gives me a clear signal when it's time to stop.

I no longer crave sweets and starches; I'm just not interested in eating them. I've been relieved of my obsession with food. Instead, I have peace of mind like I've never known before. I still have weight to release, but I have no doubt it will eventually happen because I'm not fighting with my body anymore. I'm at peace with what I need to do. I can literally feel inflammation leaving my body, and I'm grateful—so grateful.

I have a lot more energy now, and the anxiety and depression I once felt have vanished. I will always have Hashimoto's, and I am still very sensitive to cold, but that's one of the reasons I live in St. George, Utah—because it's so nice and warm! I keep my pool warm and work out vigorously six days a week. It's a total sanctuary for me.

There's a saying: when the student is ready, the teacher shows up. When I felt like I was at the end of my rope, I was at that point. I was ready to be taught. The truth for my body could be presented to me and I would listen. This healthcare provider had the truth I desperately needed. He showed up at just the right time, and it's been a joyful, peaceful, and incredible journey ever since. I am grateful for the heavenly help that helps me stay on my path to healing.

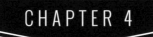

Trust Your Instincts

Jessica's Story

Jessica is a 31-year-old stay-at-home mom who enjoys her busy routine and thrives on the responsibilities involved in caring for her family and home. This is an astounding feat because, not long ago, Jessica was bedridden with no hope of ever feeling better. No one knew what was wrong—healthcare provider after healthcare provider failed to find the cause of her illness, and no medication or therapy provided relief. Jessica feared for her life.

> "I never told anyone how bad I felt because I knew from experience it wouldn't get me anywhere. I didn't want to complain. I was doing everything I could to find an answer, but no one could find anything wrong with me. I began to question myself, and started wondering if I was just crazy. I didn't want anyone else to wonder, too, so I kept my illness to myself."

Have you ever considered why you get up every day and do all the things you have to do, even when you don't feel well? If you have, you might say something like, "I do it for my kids," or, "It's just part of life. You have to take the good times with the bad." For a lot of people, I think there's also something more—a sense that their lives are on a path of improvement, a hope for the future, even on the worst days, and confidence that things are going to get better.

That hope and confidence—those are things I never had.

Ever since I can remember, I lived with the belief that things weren't going to get *better*, they were going to get *worse*. As a child, I'd look at my parents and grandparents and think I'd never live that long. I'd never have a full life because sooner or later—probably sooner—my body is just going to shut down.

I constantly felt sick when I was young, but I didn't know what was wrong. I remember being very young and doctors telling my mom I had food allergies. She'd take me off certain foods for a while, but I would ask again and again for things I shouldn't have. Eventually, my mom would cave and let me eat whatever I wanted.

I was an active kid, and was diagnosed with ADHD. Looking back, I think my problems were a result of my food sensitivities. I struggled in school: I never got good grades, and it was impossible for me to concentrate, no matter how hard I tried. I felt dumb.

If there was a flu or cold bug going around, I got it—and I got it twice as bad for twice as long. I was also constantly losing and regaining weight.

I remember being in school, eating something for lunch or a snack, and then being in so much pain I'd start to sweat. I'd run into the bathroom, hide in a stall, and take off layer after layer of clothing. I was terrified of being caught, but I felt like my body was on fire. My hair would get

Redd Flag

Jessica suffered from common autoimmune symptoms since she was a child. Frequent sickness is a common first symptom of autoimmune conditions. Patients often get sick easily and stay sick longer.[12]

The second common symptom is food reactions. Research has shown that autoimmune responses can be correlated with a loss of integrity of the intestinal membrane barrier. Patients start absorbing certain proteins into the blood stream that they shouldn't. A cascade of intestinal inflammation and inflammatory cytokines follows.[13]

soaked with sweat. Eventually, I'd go back to class and everyone would just stare at me, wondering why my hair was wet and what I'd been doing. I had no idea what was wrong with me.

I complained to my parents about my horrible stomach pain, and my mom took me to doctor after doctor. It was the same story, over and over. "We can't find anything wrong. Let's treat you for an ulcer," they'd say. Or, "Nothing is wrong, so let's try treating you for a parasite." I was given a different medication every time.

One time, I remember going in for a follow-up visit after—yet again—the medication didn't help. The doctor asked me to leave the room, but I could hear what he was saying through the door: he told my mom I was a hypochondriac, and that nothing was wrong with me. I was put on an antidepressant.

My mom wanted to believe me, but she eventually gave up. (After all, the medical professionals couldn't find anything wrong with me!) Once that happened, I was no longer just sick and miserable—I was sick and miserable and alone. When I realized nobody was going to help me and nothing was going to change, I stopped complaining.

Until my mid-twenties, my stomach hurt every time I ate. I struggled through the pain, convincing myself it wasn't really that bad. I reminded myself that there were other people out there who have had to overcome far worse ills in life.

I was low on iron when I went away for college, and my healthcare provider told me to eat as much iron-rich foods as I could. Since I had a hard time getting anything in my stomach, fortified cereals were pretty much all I ate during my entire freshman year. I suppose I thought of the cereal like some sort of good luck charm to keep my life going.

At the end of that year, I was on vacation with a friend, driving, and my vision began to blur. My body felt tingly, I was numb on one side, and I felt like my system was shutting down. I was certain my luck had finally run out. I went straight to the ER. In the emergency room I said to my friend, "Call my family. I'm dying."

The hospital performed extensive blood work, and my red and white blood cell counts were really off. They did a biopsy of my colon and diagnosed me with Celiac disease. Despite this news, I was so thankful to be alive.

I immediately went on a strict, gluten-free diet and saw improvements pretty quickly. My problems didn't go away, but I was relieved to finally start feeling better. I didn't get sick as often, and the intense pain and sweating I'd suffered with for years faded away. Unfortunately, going gluten free didn't get rid of all my symptoms.

I got married and started having kids, and I could no longer function—I was so sluggish and tired. I couldn't maintain my energy. I was eating a healthy diet and being careful to eat nutritious food, but I was still extremely fatigued and barely had the energy to get through the day.

As a new wife and a mom with young babies, I needed more energy. Coffee wasn't enough, no matter how much I drank. Eventually, I started taking caffeinated diet pills that gave me the boost I needed to get through the day. I ended up taking that stuff for ten years.

Imagine this: you're a mom with a baby and a toddler and the only way you can get through the day is by going to the drug store to buy diet pills. I was so embarrassed. I shouldn't have been taking them—I knew they weren't good for me—but I felt like I had no choice. I wanted to stop before my husband found out—before I did serious harm to my already sick body. I tried going to holistic health practitioners for help, but nothing worked. They all just tried to treat the symptoms, so no one ever put the pieces together and diagnosed the underlying cause of my illness. I ended up going back to the stimulants time and time again, just to get by.

I'd go to a doctor and say, "I have no energy. I never feel rested." They'd guess what pills might make me feel better and try it. Anti-depressants, iron supplements, and sleeping pills—nothing worked. I tried holistic therapies: energy tapping, foot reflexology, and anything that might make me feel better. You name it, I tried it. I was open to anything, but there was never a solution.

Not surprisingly, all of this had a terrible impact on my marriage. It was rough. I was getting sicker and sicker, and I wasn't able to take care of my kids or the house or handle any of my responsibilities. My husband would come home frustrated every night; at the same time, he was worried. He watched my health decline. The fact that I was not making any progress with my health was a huge strain on our marriage. I just couldn't fix it.

Things hit rock bottom after I had my third baby. I never bounced back. I never felt good, or healthy. I was constantly fighting one virus or another and had zero energy. I couldn't function. I knew all mothers are tired to an extent, but this was way more extreme than lack of sleep and postpartum blues.

I never told anyone how bad I felt because I knew from experience it wouldn't get me anywhere. I didn't want to complain. I was doing everything I could to find an answer, but no one could find anything wrong with me. I began to question myself, and started wondering if I was just crazy. I didn't want anyone else to wonder, too, so I kept my illness to myself.

I was so desperate for a solution that I underwent an extreme detox in the summer of 2011. That was the beginning of a major change for me. Seeing what came out of my body confirmed the fact that I was incredibly sick. The detox flushed metals and parasites out of my body. Pretty disgusting.

The practitioner I worked with said all of my organs were so strained that she couldn't understand how I hadn't been diagnosed with a heart condition. Her words validated what I'd felt all along: my system was shutting down. My body was so toxic that I was dying.

After the detox, frightened by the extent and degree of my illness, I made strict changes to my diet. I cut out corn, and I never ate sugar. This seemed to help sometimes, but I'd always crash. I'd have a good day and think, "Okay, I feel good. I want to have more kids!" Then I'd have ten bad days and realize I couldn't even take care of the kids I already had. I never knew how I was going to feel.

In January of 2012, with little remaining hope, I visited yet another doctor. This time, things were radically different. Instead of being handed a prescription and sent on my way to "wait and see," I was diagnosed with Hashimoto's disease. I was so relieved, I cried. For the first time ever, I thought I'd found the answer—maybe I'd even found a solution.

The doctor put me on medication, and my symptoms became even worse. Suddenly, I went from feeling like I'd finally found an answer to being more frightened and discouraged than ever. I was so sick that I couldn't get out of bed for a month.

My healthcare practitioner was at a complete loss as to how to help me. She said, "I don't know why your body isn't reacting well, and I don't know what to do with you." I had spent thousands of dollars on tests and treatment, but I didn't feel better and she didn't know what to do. She didn't give up on me, but she made it clear I wasn't a typical patient and wasn't reacting the way she'd expected and hoped I would.

I finally decided I couldn't take it any longer, and stopped taking the medication my practitioner had prescribed. I told her I would rather die than lay in bed, feeling the way I did. I meant it.

> ## Redd Flag
> Low thyroid patients are often put on a thyroid hormone, which they may need, but this does not address the problem causing the low thyroid to begin with. In such cases, the patient's condition is unlikely to improve over time.[14]

At this point, I was so low and so sick that I was desperate. I finally opened up, and told my family how I was feeling. I told them I was hopeless and devastated, and asked them to help me. For ten years, no one had realized just how sick I really was. How could they? I hadn't told them. I'd even hidden the extent of my illness from my husband.

Maybe I just had to get that low before I would ask for help, but once I did, everything started falling into place.

It wasn't long after I decided to open up that another opportunity came along—one that changed everything. A healthcare professional who works with "tough" Hashimoto's cases appeared on the TV show my sister hosts. My sister, who now knew I was desperately sick, approached him and asked if there was anything he could do to help me. He told her to send me in to see him.

I was nervous when I went in for my appointment—I was almost afraid to have too much hope. I'd lived with health failure after health failure, but what happened during that appointment was amazing: I knew immediately I'd found what I'd been searching for my entire life.

I recognized a major difference in his approach to my condition. He not only listened as I described my symptoms, he actually understood what I described—and he believed me! Then he took the time to explain what was likely happening in my body, how he could help, and why.

I immediately quit the diet I'd been on to focus on my new care plan. This new practitioner's approach was to avoid foods my body was intolerant to in order to calm the inflammation in my body. Side by side, the two diets were very different, and I knew

Redd Flag

Foods often play a big role in flaring up Hashimoto's disease and other autoimmune responses,[15] but it's not the only factor that will cause a flare. Patients typically have multiple physiological triggers that increase the autoimmune response in addition to dietary and environmental triggers.[16]

the program I had been on simply wasn't enough. I needed to do far more than eliminate common food allergens—my body needed to heal.

I started feeling so much better once I understood and could control my autoimmunity and the triggers that caused it to flare. My energy skyrocketed. I'd always crashed at 4:00 pm and would need to take another diet pill to boost me through the next six hours. On my new care plan, I was awake and alert with energy until 7:00 pm. Then 9:00 pm. Finally, I didn't need diet pills to get through the day!

As I worked with this practitioner, I found answers to questions I'd had my whole life. I already knew I had Celiac disease and Hashimoto's, but there was more. Extensive testing revealed

> ## Redd Flag
> When a patient has inflammatory markers that are drastically out of range, it's important to start strategies that will have anti-inflammatory effects.[2] This provides for a better and faster outcome as other imbalances throughout the body are addressed.

the cause of my inflammation: my immune system was attacking my brain, my nerves, the lining of my stomach, and even my skin. Not great news, I know, but I was relieved. I finally felt validated instead of crazy—there was a real, verified reason for all the pain, suffering, and sickness I'd endured for so many years.

I've gotten sick twice since I started my care plan. Both times happened when I "cheated" and ate something I knew I shouldn't. I learned the hard way the difference between sticking to my diet versus straying. Since then, I've stuck to the foods I know are good for my body. I have a choice to eat what looks good and feel bad, or eat what I should and feel good—and I know how I want to feel!

Health has become a family affair—my mother and four sisters are all going to the clinic that changed my life. As for my husband, he's grateful I finally feel good. He noticed when everything started going more smoothly at home—the house was clean again, the kids were happier, and things were more organized. The wife he wanted was appearing before his eyes.

> ## Redd Flag
> Often, when a family member has a thyroid problem other family members will have it too. If it is caused by autoimmunity, family members may have different types of autoimmune conditions.[17] We see families where each person has a different autoimmune disease.

All three of my children have autoimmune diseases, and they experience many of the same health struggles I did at a young age. They won't have to suffer, because I understand their needs—I am empowered to help them have better lives than I did.

My life is now filled with hope, freedom, and choices I never felt I really had. I wanted to have more kids after my third baby, but I had written it off because my health was so bad. At my last health care visit, I asked my practitioner about the possibility of pregnancy. He said I'm probably healthier now than I was when I had my first three children, and he thinks my body and my baby would be just fine!

I came out of this experience knowing I have a choice in how my future plays out. I no longer feel helpless, isolated and afraid. Before, my poor health controlled my entire life. I don't live like that anymore— my life is no longer centered on sickness, it revolves around what I love!

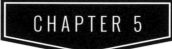

CHAPTER 5

Hope and a Family After Multiple Miscarriages

Shannon's Story

Shannon, a registered nurse, knows a lot about low thyroid and the heartbreaking impact it can have on women eager to start a family. Some of her knowledge comes from her professional training as an RN; much of it is from firsthand experience.

The symptoms associated with hypothyroidism are often frustrating and debilitating, and can even be life threatening. As Shannon learned, they can also destroy a couple's dreams of having children. Health problems associated with Hashimoto's disease turned what should be one of the most beautiful and natural experiences a woman can have into a nightmare for Shannon—not once, but twice. If you're a low thyroid patient who's suffered one or more miscarriages, or if you're hoping for a healthy pregnancy in the future, Shannon's story contains valuable information.

◇◇◇◇◇◇◇◇◇◇◇◇◇◇◇◇◇◇◇◇◇◇◇◇

"Losing my third child was like a confirmation of all my fears; all the darkness I saw in the world came to fruition. I started to feel paranoid–to believe I was doomed to suffer for the rest of my life. I was put on anxiety medication in addition to the antidepressants, but it made me even more exhausted than I already was."

◇◇◇◇◇◇◇◇◇◇◇◇◇◇◇◇◇◇◇◇◇◇◇◇

My health problems didn't begin until I was in my early thirties. In May of 2010, I began gaining weight even though I ate a healthy diet and exercised regularly. I felt tired every day, even after a lot of sleep. When I began to experience insomnia, that fatigue turned into chronic exhaustion.

I started struggling with anxiety and depression. I worried about everything—paying the bills on time, my patients at work, and even the weather! Although I'd been a happy person all my life, I started feeling a dark sense of dread about the day ahead and the future. I was consumed with negativity about my life and everything around me.

All of these symptoms felt foreign; I knew something wasn't right, so I went to my general practitioner for help. She ran blood tests, and diagnosed me with Hashimoto's disease. As it happened, my GP had Hashimoto's herself, and was very familiar with it. I was hopeful I'd start feeling better soon.

I started taking thyroid medication. Although my symptoms improved a bit, I still had a general feeling of being unwell. I felt tired every day. It was as if I was dragging myself through everything I had to do—get up, shower, dress, get to work, and make it through the morning. At lunchtime, I would wonder how I could possibly get through the afternoon. Then, as the day wore on, I'd daydream about how good it would feel to finally get into bed. I dreaded the time I'd have to spend eating dinner and trying to stay awake for the sake of my husband.

I still had a good deal of anxiety and depression, and I also started having dizzy spells. Life had once been fun, but at the time it was torture. Nothing made me feel good. Nothing was rewarding.

My mind was foggy, and my memory was suffering. I'd walk into a room and then forget what I needed or why I was there. I'd be talking to patients and draw a blank; I'd forget everything they'd just said. It wasn't long before I ended up in my patients' shoes—feeling like medical professionals weren't listening to me.

That year, my husband and I started trying to get pregnant. We'd planned to have kids, and I didn't see any reason to put it off. I guess I was hoping a new baby would turn things around for me—give me a fresh start. I learned in December that I had conceived, and was elated. Even better, I was expecting twins! I still didn't feel great, but I pushed my health problems to the back of my mind because I was so thrilled to be pregnant.

In January of 2011, I lost my babies. Suddenly, my mental and physical health spiraled out of control. The loss of the twins made my anxiety and depression a hundred times worse. I cried constantly. I felt more miserable and alone than I had in my entire life; I was a complete mess. I did my best to hide how terrible I felt because the last thing I wanted to do after our loss was worry my husband.

My outlook was bleak, to say the least. I couldn't sleep, and I didn't feel well. I was exhausted. Every day was one huge chore after another; even basic tasks like house cleaning required major effort. I felt like a zombie. It didn't matter to me what I did because it all felt the same— like a huge burden I could barely handle.

My doctor put me on antidepressants. Like the thyroid medication, the antidepressants helped a little, but I still experienced anxiety and depression.

I struggled through the first half of 2011. I got by, but barely. In the summer of that year, I got pregnant again. My hopes soared, but I was a lot more skeptical about my ability to carry a baby to term. I felt like I was walking on eggshells, and my anxiety was off the charts. I wanted this baby so badly! I talked to my OB and GP about my fears and concerns, and they both said the same thing: "There is nothing wrong. Don't worry."

The first week in October, I had my second miscarriage. I fell into a deep depression and experienced even more intense anxiety. Losing my third child was like a confirmation of all my fears; all the darkness I saw in the world came to fruition. I started to feel paranoid—to believe I was doomed to suffer for the rest of my life. I was put on anxiety medication in addition to the antidepressants, but it made me even more exhausted than I already was.

I knew that my miscarriages exacerbated my depression and anxiety. It was a vicious cycle I wanted to break, but the medications didn't do much good. I know a lot about pharmaceuticals, and I knew that everything that should have helped me had failed.

I went back to my healthcare practitioners to try to figure out why I was losing my babies. They did all kinds of tests. They evaluated my uterus for malformations, but found nothing. They tested my hormones, but couldn't identify a problem. When I'd tell anyone at my healthcare providers' offices how I felt, they seemed to just ignore what I said. Instead of giving me answers, my doctors told me, "You're fine. There is nothing specific causing your miscarriages and we're sure you'll have a baby some day." In their eyes, they had given me a clean bill of health. They couldn't find the problem, so they didn't want to keep searching.

Considering how much I'd suffered and how badly I was feeling, you can imagine how frustrating this was. On one hand, I wanted to believe that I was healthy; on the other, I knew a third miscarriage would take a huge toll on both my husband and me. In my gut, I knew something just wasn't right. There had to be something more to it.

I went to see different general practitioners and an endocrinologist, but it was all the same story. They ran the same tests over and over and based their treatment on my hormone levels. They didn't care how I felt; they cared about numbers. They used the numbers to make medication adjustments, but they never tried to find an underlying problem—the true cause of all my symptoms.

When I was initially diagnosed with Hashimoto's I thought, "Okay, I have hypothyroidism. I'll take medication and feel better." That is what I knew from my experience in the medical profession. That's the extent of it. I wasn't taught that Hashimoto's was something different from low thyroid—that it is in fact an autoimmune disease—and I know my health practitioners weren't taught about it either. Once I realized thyroid medication wasn't going to improve my health and allow me to carry my babies to term, I began to do my own research.

When I started reading *Why Do I Still Have Thyroid Symptoms? When My Lab Tests Are Normal* by Datis Kharrazian, my first thought was, "Oh, my gosh, this is me! This is exactly what's going on in my body!" I was so blown away by this doctor's knowledge about Hashimoto's and his unique approach to its management that I brought a copy of the book to my practitioner. I felt so strongly that this book was about me, and that this approach was vital to my wellness and my ability to have a child.

My healthcare provider wasn't enthused about the book's recommendations, but I sure was. I immediately made some of the dietary changes he recommended by limiting my consumption of gluten, but that was the extent of what I could do on my own. There's a lot of testing and personalized care involved in his approach, and each patient has to be managed properly. The full protocol requires supplements you can't just go buy at the health food store or order online. I didn't have the knowledge or expertise to heal myself, but at least I'd learned that help was possible with the right approach.

After doing more research, I found a healthcare professional who had experience working with Kharrazian's protocol. Luckily, his office was close by. I burst into tears, I was so happy! At that moment, I knew I was going to get the care I so desperately needed and wanted.

My new practitioner ran more tests than I'd ever had. When the results came back and I went in to meet with him, he said, "You're really sick. It must be so hard for you; I bet you rarely feel well." It was such a huge relief to know this healthcare provider understood! He didn't think I was crazy; he knew how sick I was, and he understood how unwell I was feeling.

Even more importantly, this provider recognized that the loss of my babies was weighing heavily on me. He told me he thought he knew why I had miscarried, and that he could help me try to have the baby my husband and I wanted so badly. He said we would address all the inflammation in my body, and that my hormones needed to be balanced. He truly wanted to help me.

Being a nurse, I recognized immediately that this healthcare provider's approach was different. He was extremely thorough, and checked my hormone levels through saliva testing instead of relying only on blood tests. This type of testing is a lot more accurate and gives a more complete picture of what's really going on, which is exactly what was necessary in my case.

No one had ever tested my testosterone levels, and it turned out they were elevated for my age and gender. This resulted in insulin resistance. Even though I'm not diabetic, it was another important piece of the big picture.

I'm convinced that customized care plans using this approach can help Hashimoto's patients. Mine started out with a pretty strict diet, and I took several different supplements to address the imbalances all the tests had revealed. I noticed a difference in my energy level within about two weeks! Before I started working with my new practitioner, my energy level was at a two or three. Then it felt like a five. As time went by, it went up to six and seven.

I began sleeping better almost right away. In the past, even though I was exhausted at bedtime, I'd lay awake all night unable to sleep. Falling asleep and getting a good night's rest was a totally new and refreshing experience.

I also started to lose weight, and it happened in a fascinating way. The numbers on the scale

Redd Flag

Women with insulin resistance and/or PCOS are more likely to suffer a miscarriage than their peers.[18]

Research has shown a strong correlation between PCOS and autoimmune low thyroid. Researchers found that 42% of patients suffering with PCOS had hypoechoic tissue typical of an autoimmune thyroid condition, and that almost 27% of patients suffering with PCOS had thyroid antibodies.[19]

If you have infertility or problems carrying a baby full term, it's a good idea to have these two conditions ruled out immediately.

didn't move much, but my body composition totally changed; I looked like I had lost fifteen pounds even though I had only lost five. I was building lean muscle, so I looked better and felt great. The anxiety and depression I'd struggled with for so long seemed to just fade away. It was a complete transformation—unlike anything I've ever experienced.

I learned how to recognize my body's cues when I react to something I eat or drink, and I learned how to help myself feel better if I have a flare up. I still really struggle with gluten. I'm not allergic to it, but it affects my energy level tremendously; I feel completely tired and wiped out any time I consume gluten.

I became pregnant about six months into my care plan, and I had no complications throughout my pregnancy. I felt great, and I was able to enjoy the miraculous experience of pregnancy. I didn't really even worry about miscarrying—the difference in my health was that huge.

My son, Bridger, is six months old now, and I'm back to working full time. Do I feel tired or exhausted these days? You bet, but it's a different kind of tired. I'm happy now, and there's a reason I'm tired at the end of the day—it's because I'm living a full life as a mom, a wife, and a busy nurse! I cherish my health every single day, just like I cherish my son.

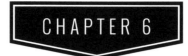

CHAPTER 6

Being Sick Is Not a "Normal Part of Aging"

Edye's Story

What happens when older people are stricken with debilitating health problems that don't involve obviously terminal diseases, like cancer or heart disease? As Edye learned, a practitioner's dismissive attitude can have devastating consequences.

Not even at early retirement age, Edye was overwhelmed with pain, exhaustion, and other serious health conditions. Although she was unable to function, she was told time and time again that what she was experiencing was "just a normal part of aging."

Willing to do anything to get well, but with no help or hope in sight, Edye prepared to say goodbye to her beloved grandson. She even arranged her own funeral.

◇◇◇◇◇◇◇◇◇◇◇◇◇◇◇◇◇◇◇◇◇◇◇

"I'd never been depressed in my life, but with the changes in my health, my appearance, the pain, and the fact that I could no longer do everything I was accustomed to doing, I knew I couldn't go on much longer. My body deteriorated so quickly that I was sure I was going to die."

◇◇◇◇◇◇◇◇◇◇◇◇◇◇◇◇◇◇◇◇◇◇◇

My health problems first began when I was in my late fifties. I've worked as a property manager for decades, so I was always pretty good at handling long hours and stress. I ate healthy foods and exercised every day, and, for the most part, I was the epitome of good health. Then, it was as if everything changed overnight.

I was working out of town to do a turnaround on a challenging property. My job was to get the property operating efficiently and profitably, and I was working long, long hours. I was accustomed to putting a lot of time and energy into my work, but something was different this time. At the end of my day I would return to my temporary apartment, collapse on the sofa, and fall asleep. Sometimes I'd sleep there all night, and sometimes I'd wake up and have dinner and go straight to bed. Either way, this exhaustion wasn't normal for me.

While I was still out of town, I went to donate at a blood drive. After they pricked my finger they said I needed to see a doctor right away. It was pretty scary, especially because I was away from home. I asked around the office to find out where I should go for medical care, and chose a practitioner based on those recommendations.

It felt like it took forever to get in for an appointment, and when I finally did the practitioner's biggest concern seemed to be following a script! Nobody asked, "What's wrong with this person? Why does this seemingly healthy woman suddenly need so much sleep?" Instead I heard, "When was your last mammogram?" and, "Have you had a colonoscopy?"

They did a blood test, which showed that my thyroid was a little low. The doctor gave me a prescription for 25mcgs of thyroid hormone, and told me I'd have to take it the rest of my life. Over the next six years, those 25mcgs turned into 137mcgs and I felt worse and worse instead of better.

What I experienced may be hard to understand unless you've

> ## Redd Flag
>
> If your doctor regularly increases the dose of your thyroid medications, it's important to figure out what is causing the lack of thyroid hormone production. Often (but not always), it is because the patient's thyroid is being attacked and destroyed by the immune system.[5] Calming down the autoimmunity is crucial to minimize tissue destruction. [20]

been through it yourself. I had extreme fatigue to the point where it was all I could do to stay awake long enough to work. I developed excruciating pain—I had so much pain in my knees and legs that I could barely walk. I couldn't even stand up out of a chair; I had to pull myself up holding on to something or somebody, and once I was finally standing it took time to adjust to the pain before I could move. Going up or down stairs took forever. I researched chair lifts for my house—it had gotten that bad.

It wasn't just pain and exhaustion that made working nearly impossible; I also had gastrointestinal problems. I couldn't think clearly. I itched constantly, all over my body. I started gaining weight that I just could not lose. My face was breaking out non-stop. My hair started falling out. I was feeling more and more depressed.

I'd never been depressed in my life, but with the changes in my health, my appearance, the pain, and the fact that I could no longer do everything I was accustomed to doing, I knew I couldn't go on much longer. My body deteriorated so quickly that I was sure I was going to die.

The thing is, I was too young for all these health problems. I visited multiple health advisors and practices, and heard the same things over and over. I would describe the extreme pain in my legs, and they wouldn't even look at my knees. "You're getting older," they'd say, "It's probably a little arthritis." It was the same thing with my hair falling out, the itching, and the exhaustion. Again and again I heard "Just take your new dose of medicine and see how you feel."

> ## Redd Flag
> If you have Hashimoto's disease and you're experiencing pain, one important thing to check for is rheumatoid arthritis,[9(p.168)] which can be tricky to diagnose. Another potential cause of pain is the inflammatory cytokines that are produced in Hashimoto's low thyroid patients. This can create a lot of swelling and water retention along with pain in the joints and muscles.[21]

When I started gaining weight and talked to a doctor about it, she said, "It's harder when you're older. Don't eat fried foods, pizza, or dessert." I hadn't eaten fried foods in 40 years! Yes, I had pizza or dessert once in a while, but really? Having something sweet after a meal on occasion was causing major weight gain? I didn't think so.

I saw three different health practitioners for my weight gain and inability to lose a pound. The only thing I heard was, "Try the latest fill-in-the-blank diet. You're older; you have to watch what you eat. Deal with it."

It made me angry at the time, and thinking about it now is infuriating. Just because you're getting older or you have low thyroid doesn't mean you can't have a quality life! It doesn't mean you can't do anything—that you can't walk! There are plenty of older people who are quite active and feel great, and I knew this. I wasn't buying into what I was hearing, but there was nothing I could do except keep going back, keep searching for something else, and keep hoping someone would listen.

I pushed hard for answers, I did a lot of research, and I kept telling my health advisors I needed more extensive testing. I believed I had inflammation and other hormonal imbalances—that something more was going on. I told my practitioner at the time that I needed to find out what was wrong with me once and for all, and I was willing to do whatever it took to do so.

That practitioner actually discouraged me from seeing a thyroid specialist. She said the testing I was talking about was something they didn't do locally, and that even if they could do it, it was very expensive. I wanted to ask her if she would be willing to suffer like I was—or even die—because of inconvenience or cost.

At that point, I knew I was dying. I could literally feel my whole body shutting down. I was getting up at night and vomiting for no reason. For days on end, I couldn't regulate myself well enough to eat anything at all. Deep inside, I knew nobody could feel as bad as I felt and be as sick as I was and live for long.

I was preparing to die. After that last discouraging conversation with my health practitioner, I planned my funeral—I decided what I wanted to wear, how I wanted the service to be, and where I wanted to be buried.

My grandson has always been the absolute love of my life—I adopted and raised him, so we have a mother-son relationship. He's almost 24 now, and lives in a converted apartment in my basement, but he'll always be my baby. Once I got to the point where I knew I was dying, I started leaving notes for him so he'd know where things were and what bills needed to be paid and when. I tried to think of everything he might need to know about our home so he would be prepared when I was gone.

Of course, I never let anyone in on what I was thinking or feeling. I didn't want my grandson or my friends to worry about something they couldn't do anything about, and I didn't want them to know how depressed I was. I didn't want my bosses to know what was going on because I was afraid they'd think I wasn't able to work anymore and lay me off from the job I love. I was very careful to put on a brave face all the time.

Then, I was told about a health practitioner who helped people suffering with severe symptoms of low thyroid from all over the world— people just like me. I jotted down the information about him and went online to look up his clinic. I thought to myself, "Okay, this could be legit, or it could be one of those 'take this pill and lose five pounds tonight' scams." It was hard to imagine that anyone could be serious when they claimed to be able to help people who are as sick as I was. I had to do research before I would even consider that this might be the real deal.

Finally, I figured I really had nothing to lose. I called and made an appointment for a phone interview. I was in so much pain at the time—so unable to function—that I couldn't even make the 25-mile drive to visit the office in person. As we began to talk on the day of my appointment, I knew this was a very different type of health care.

First of all, the practitioner wanted to know everything about what I'd experienced—all of my symptoms and all that I'd been through. When I finished, he wasn't dismissive. I didn't hear, "You're just getting older." I could tell this man was actually listening to what I was saying and truly wanted to help.

The practitioner did the testing I'd been begging other practitioners to do. He explained that the type of care he offered low thyroid patients wasn't right for everyone, and it wasn't going to be a "take your medicine and see how you feel" deal. I had to be committed to getting better and willing to follow his recommendations or there was really no way this care plan could help me. I was more than ready—I'd been willing to do whatever it would take to get better for years!

I got started with the tests, and it turned out my hunches were right: I had extensive inflammation and imbalances throughout my body—extreme gluten intolerance and other sensitivities and digestive problems. I made dietary changes and took the herbal supplements the practitioner suggested, and the results were incredible. I wouldn't believe the change my body went through if I hadn't experienced it firsthand.

To start with, my knees and legs were almost 100% better within a week. I could walk! I could go up and down stairs. I could stand up out of a chair and sit down by myself. I was out of my mind with relief. The

> ## Redd Flag
> Low thyroid and Hashimoto's patients have to work just as hard as their practitioners to gain the best outcomes. There are many physiological triggers that we can address to drastically help the patient improve,[22] but there are also dietary and lifestyle triggers that the patients must address themselves.

excruciating itching I'd suffered with for years went away. My hair stopped falling out. The gas and bloating stopped. I didn't have to throw up in the middle of the night. All of that went away.

I had stopped putting foods into my body that caused it to react violently, and my inflammation subsided. The right supplements calmed things down. I started getting well.

The results have been amazing, but there's more to it than simply feeling good again. The practitioner taught me how to watch what is happening in my body and understand how I react to foods. He gave me the tools I needed to take care of myself. It's a completely different approach from anything I've ever encountered in medical care.

Today, I have a lifestyle I know I can live with that will support my health for the rest of my life. I no longer have cravings for foods that don't agree with my body—I don't care about gluten or sugar. I don't miss a thing! I've lost over 51 pounds so far. I'm not on a weight loss program, but I'm delighted to have shed all the extra weight I'd gained over the years when I was so sick.

It's been one and a half years since I first started working with my present practitioner, and I'm doing great. I'm still on thyroid medication and I know I will be the rest of my life, but my dose is down to 88mcgs and holding steady. I feel fantastic, and I'm confident I can keep feeling this way for many years to come.

I'm sure a lot of people would tell me that at my age I've already lived my life—why don't I just face facts when it comes to aging? Well, my life is not over, and it wasn't meant to be over the whole time I was literally dying. I have so much more life to live, and age has nothing to do with it.

I would be dead, lying in my grave right now in a dress I picked out three years ago, if it wasn't for my new healthcare plan. Instead, I'm living a life I love and enjoying my grandson, my work, and my friends. All it took was someone to listen and give me the chance and the tools to learn how to take care of my own health. That's what we all really need, no matter what our age.

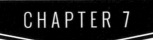

CHAPTER 7

Redefining "Diet"

Leslie H.'s Story

Leslie loves to travel and thrives on the challenges of her career as director of operations for a financial services group. She recently took an exciting two-week trip to Europe, traveling to countries she had dreamed of visiting for years.

Not long ago, Leslie's health was so poor that she would never have made that trip. Her Hashimoto's disease had caused extreme fatigue, weight gain, and debilitating headaches—just making it through the day was a struggle. By finding a practitioner who understood her condition, learning about Hashimoto's, and committing to staying healthy, Leslie has taken control of her health. Her thyroid struggles no longer prevent her from living her life to the fullest.

◇◇◇◇◇◇◇◇◇◇◇◇◇◇◇◇◇◇◇◇◇◇◇◇

"When none of the tests or consultations shed light on my weight gain, my doctor finally admitted she was at a bit of a loss. She basically threw her hands up in the air and said, 'I don't know what to tell you.' She didn't exactly accuse me of lying, but she did say, 'If you're doing everything you say you're doing, there's no reason why you shouldn't lose weight.'"

◇◇◇◇◇◇◇◇◇◇◇◇◇◇◇◇◇◇◇◇◇◇◇◇

When I was younger, I could always take off any weight I put on. Then, three or so years ago, around the time I turned forty, my weight suddenly became a huge problem. I began to gain excessively. You know how uncomfortable you feel when you put on ten pounds over the holidays? Well, I gained 50 pounds in just 5 months.

As soon as I noticed I was gaining weight, I started to diet and exercise like crazy. When I say I dieted, I don't mean I casually cut back on my food intake. I followed strict calorie guidelines and I focused on eating healthy foods like veggies, fruits, lean meat, and whole grains. I didn't eat sweets or fried foods, and didn't "cheat." Still, I couldn't lose a pound. Even more frightening, I kept gaining.

I was shocked at how quickly my body was changing. First my clothes got tight, and then they didn't fit at all; I'd buy a new set of clothes, and within a month they were too small for me.

When people diet without seeing results, they can often pinpoint why. They might feel annoyed when the dial on the scale hasn't moved for a week, but if they think back they'll remember adding extra butter to the veggies, snacking on a handful of cookies, or grabbing an extra helping of mashed potatoes. In my case, despite doing everything in my power to control my diet, I couldn't lose the weight and I couldn't figure out why.

At the time, I was under the care of my regular family doctor. She ran a lot of tests to try to figure out what was going on, and I was sure she'd be able to help me. I also went to a nutritionist to try to find anything I might be overlooking. I had my basal metabolic rate tested, but it showed nothing unusual—I had no explanation for why I couldn't stop gaining weight.

When none of the tests or consultations shed light on my weight gain, my doctor finally admitted she was at a bit of a loss. She basically threw her hands up in the air and said, "I don't know what to tell you." She didn't exactly accuse me of lying, but she did say, "If you're doing everything you say you're doing, there's no reason why you shouldn't lose weight." I'd already been discouraged; learning there wasn't a "medical" answer to my problem made me feel even more afraid and out of control of my own health.

At this point, I started getting severe headaches. The pain began in the morning as I was getting ready for work, and intensified throughout the day. I could barely function if I didn't take something, so I took acetaminophen or ibuprofen every day at lunchtime. They barely touched the pain, but I could get through the rest of the day if I took twice the normal dose. At night, I would fall asleep in pain, knowing I'd wake up with the same headache. I lived with this every single day.

Not long after the headaches started, I began to feel extremely tired. No matter how hard I tried to rest and get more sleep, I was always too exhausted to do anything in the evenings. It was all I could do to make it through dinner before falling asleep on the couch. I knew I should exercise, but it was impossible; taking even one step made me feel like collapsing.

I knew I had all the symptoms of a thyroid problem—and my practitioner agreed—but my thyroid tests came back normal.

I had experienced thyroid problems in the past. In 2005, about five years before I started gaining the weight, I was diagnosed with a hyperactive thyroid. I had been having heart palpitations at the time, and ended up seeing an endocrinologist who diagnosed me with hyperthyroid. I took medication for about six months, at which point testing showed I was no longer hyperthyroid. My thyroid seemed to be functioning normally again, and my practitioner believed that whatever had been going on with my thyroid had been resolved.

Eight years later, in January of 2013 after my thyroid tests had come back normal, my health practitioner left her practice. I had to find a new doctor and start at the beginning—explaining my symptoms and history all over again. By then, my weight had climbed to 252 pounds. This was a huge amount of weight for me, and I continued to feel awful.

My new healthcare practitioner ran tests, including a thyroid antibody test. At the end of January 2013, she diagnosed me with Hashimoto's disease. She told me I had to start taking medicine because eventually the disease would kill off my thyroid. It hadn't progressed that far, but I needed to start taking medication as a preventive measure.

Nobody likes to hear they have a disease, right? Well, at that point

I was just relieved to find out why I felt so badly and understand why I was struggling with weight gain. I started the medication and looked forward to getting better.

As it turned out, the medication did not agree with me. I had heart palpitations and felt panicky. I told my practitioner how I was feeling, but she wasn't very concerned. I tried not to worry, but the symptoms didn't go away. It felt like my past hypothyroid symptoms and my current thyroid problems had collided; I was sicker than ever, but I kept taking the thyroid hormone.

All along, I had kept my eyes and ears open for any option that could improve my health. One day, I heard about an office that worked with people who suffered from many different symptoms specific to Hashimoto's disease. Immediately, my ears perked up. I had every symptom, and this practice claimed to be able to help. I called and made an appointment.

On the day of my consultation, the healthcare professional learned about my history and said it sounded like I was a candidate for his care. I couldn't believe my good fortune! I was used to disappointments by that time, and was afraid it was too good to be true. But, sure enough, the initial tests he ran confirmed I had Hashimoto's disease. It wasn't that my previous practitioner had been "wrong," but the care I'd received didn't fully address my particular health concerns. This clinic was highly experienced in helping people just like me.

What made the biggest impression on me when I first visited this practice was their confidence that I could feel better. This practitioner also stressed that I could learn how to take care of my own body and my own health. It was clear that I was going to have to make a lot of lifestyle changes, but the possibility of having better health shone like a light at the end of the tunnel.

My care plan was a process. I learned why I was feeling so bad, and what triggered my symptoms. The health advisors I worked with identified food sensitivities as one of my biggest problems, as is the case for many Hashimoto's patients. They were right. They also determined I had a digestive disorder, and that my body wasn't properly absorbing vitamin D. I immediately started avoiding foods that caused my immune system to flare up because the flare-ups caused my symptoms. I learned that my body can't tolerate glu-

> ## Redd Flag
> Everyone will have to avoid different foods specific to his or her sensitivities. Some patients have to avoid many foods, but in our experience this is rare. Often, patients only have to avoid a few specific foods once their condition is calmed.

ten, and that eating wheat, oats, rye, barley, rice, corn, and dairy cause me inflammation and flare-ups.

I now eat a whole food diet composed mostly of protein, beans, vegetables, and fruits. It's a pretty strict diet by most people's standards, but in my case it's absolutely essential. As an example, I learned I have a sensitivity to corn. I had eliminated it from my diet for about 45 days and was feeling good. Then, I accidentally ate something that had corn in it and immediately started throwing up. I've stayed away from corn since then.

At this point, my body has healed so much that there are probably things I avoid eating that I might be able to tolerate in small quantities. But will I start eating corn again? No way. I know I'm sensitive to it and even if I don't get sick it's simply not worth the risk for me!

What I'm eating has made a huge difference in my health, but so has *when* I eat. I know now that I was having blood sugar problems, which interfered with my ability to sleep at night, feel rested, and get through the day without overwhelming exhaustion. When I wasn't eating at the right time, I'd wake up in the middle of the night and couldn't fall back asleep. Now that I'm following my care plan, I can go to sleep without any sleep aids, and I stay asleep all night long. I know how to eat and when to eat, so my body can rest through the night. I still have some trouble with blood sugar levels if I don't eat enough, but I've learned what that means and how to avoid it, so it's something I'm able to control.

There have been so many changes in my health and my body since I started my care plan. In 2009, I'd been diagnosed with low vitamin D levels, which can contribute to some of the symptoms I'd experienced. At the time, my level was 17; to be within my ideal range, it should have been over 40. I took prescription vitamin D back then, but the highest my level ever got was 24.

After starting my care plan, my vitamin D skyrocketed. It climbed to 58 after a few months, and now it's over 70. Once my system began healing and started processing vitamin D efficiently, it made a huge difference. My body started using calories efficiently, so my appetite started to normalize. Before, my body wasn't able to use calories as energy the way it should have—it just stored everything as fat. Even though I had been on a strict diet when I first started gaining weight, I was eating the wrong foods at the wrong time and not absorbing nutrients. No wonder I had kept gaining weight and felt so tired!

My health and well-being have changed dramatically. I've gone as long as 45 days without a headache. If I do get one, I now know what to do to address it. I no longer have to start downing pain relievers and hope for the best.

As for my weight, I started to slowly lose a few pounds after starting my care plan. It wasn't much, but it sure was motivating after gaining for so long! About a month later, the pounds just started falling off. I've now lost 44 pounds, 17% body fat, and 22 inches overall. My care plan is not a weight loss program, but I'm slimming down as my body heals. My weight loss is a natural result of changing my eating habits and taking care of my body.

Today, I look and feel completely different than I did a few years ago. I had a lot of inflammation and swelling as a result of the Hashimoto's; now that it's controlled, my body is normalizing again. I lost six pounds while I was in Europe for two weeks, despite the fact that I didn't have as much control over food options most of the time.

It used to take me hours to get going in the morning, and then I only had about three or four hours where I could be productive before I crashed in the afternoon. I would typically get home from work, put on my pajamas and lay down. I didn't have much of a social life, and I didn't go shopping after work. I waited to do everything on Saturdays because I just didn't have the energy during the week. Now, I exercise after work, take a shower, go grocery shopping, and sometimes go out again to have fun! I never would have been able to do that before.

During this journey, I also gained insight into my hyperthyroid diagnosis back in 2005. My current practitioner explained that an overactive thyroid probably wasn't the underlying cause of my heart palpations. More than likely, I've had Hashimoto's all along. I now know that this disease can cause periods of both overactive and underactive thyroid—a roller coaster of both low and high TSH levels.

At the time of my test in 2005, my levels happened to be low, so the practitioner diagnosed me with hyperactive thyroid. Since my test a few months later showed that my thyroid was no longer overactive, my practitioner concluded that the problem had been resolved. In fact, my Hashimoto's was likely causing my thyroid levels to go up and down and up and down again. Whether my thyroid was hyperactive, hypoactive or "normal" just depended on where I was on the roller coaster at the time of the test.

Ultimately, I decided the thyroid medication wasn't doing anything for me—except making me agitated—and I felt more comfortable not taking it. Now, I'm off the medication and I'll

> ## Redd Flag
> Remember, never discontinue medications without consulting your prescribing physician.

have my thyroid tested every three months. If it starts to deteriorate, I can always revisit that decision. In the meantime, the medication-induced agitation has been eliminated, my health is improved, and I feel great. I'm living a whole new life today. Every one of my friends and family members notices the difference, and even my old healthcare practitioner sees I'm much healthier, more vibrant, and a lot thinner! Life is good.

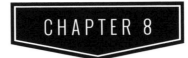

CHAPTER 8

Digestive Distress? Check Your Thyroid

Danielle's Story

Danielle is a stay-at-home mom who works as an interior designer for her husband's home building company. At 44, she's active and fit. She radiates health. Looking at her, you would never imagine she was once so sick that she lived in constant fear of being out of reach of a bathroom.

The symptoms of Danielle's thyroid condition included debilitating digestive problems and extreme anxiety. Determined to regain her health after years of illness, Danielle sought out natural, personalized care and dedicated herself to healing. Today, those symptoms no longer interfere with her busy lifestyle.

Danielle's case is a striking reminder that the symptoms of thyroid conditions and Hashimoto's disease are diverse, and that personalized care can make all the difference in the world.

◇◇◇◇◇◇◇◇◇◇◇◇◇◇◇◇◇◇◇◇◇◇◇◇◇◇◇◇

"We couldn't go anywhere as a family, and my husband ended up taking my kids to all their school functions, sports games, and friends' houses. I could barely maintain my own friendships or relax, let alone help the kids get out and have fun. My condition was a major strain on my marriage and my entire family."

◇◇◇◇◇◇◇◇◇◇◇◇◇◇◇◇◇◇◇◇◇◇◇◇◇◇◇◇

My thyroid problems began 17 years ago, at the time of my second pregnancy. My symptoms weren't severe at the time, but I did struggle with digestive problems, sluggishness, and trouble sleeping. After the birth of my second child, I just never seemed to bounce back. That time of my life marked the beginning of a decade of yo-yoing on different dosages of thyroid medication.

If you've had a thyroid problem with symptoms that won't quit, you know what I mean by yo-yoing. It's basically my expression for having my dosage upped, then lowered, then upped again—over and over. The adjustments were made according to how I was feeling and the results of my blood tests. After a while, I noticed a pattern: Whenever life became especially stressful, I'd need a different dose of thyroid medication.

In 2009, my condition became much more severe and my "normal" thyroid symptoms developed into bigger problems. Anxiety and digestive troubles were two of my biggest concerns. Whenever I ate, I'd immediately need to use the bathroom. Often, I would almost lose control of my bowels. It didn't happen after every meal, but it happened at least once a day; some days, it happened every time I ate. Whenever I ate, I had to be prepared to rush to the bathroom or risk an accident. This became a huge source of stress, anxiety, and embarrassment.

The hardest part about my condition was never knowing when or why this would happen. I couldn't pinpoint specific foods causing my digestive problems, so I couldn't stay away from triggers. It wasn't like I knew that if I ate fish, I'd have a problem, or that I would be okay as long as I didn't eat eggs—my bowels reacted to just about anything.

I've always enjoyed socializing, and I especially loved going on dates with my husband. We would go out to eat, shop, or enjoy various activities together. I quickly lost all motivation to leave the house or socialize, and there was no way I could go out to eat. It was far too stressful and embarrassing—I felt tied to the toilet.

I've always been such an outgoing person—I love people and I love traveling—but going out just wasn't worth it any more. I stopped doing the activities I had always loved.

My husband understood at first, but it didn't take long for him to feel frustrated because we couldn't do anything together. I don't believe I was ever really able to explain to him how I felt, and why I couldn't do the things we used to do.

We couldn't go anywhere as a family, and my husband ended

> ## Redd Flag
> Low thyroid and autoimmune-related health problems can have a dramatic impact on marriage and family.[23] Patients truly feel terrible that their poor health affects every aspect of their lives.

up taking my kids to all their school functions, sports games, and friends' houses. I could barely maintain my own friendships or relax, let alone help the kids get out and have fun. My condition was a major strain on my marriage and was difficult for my entire family.

I sought help from a lot of different healthcare practitioners. I was told more than once that I might have irritable bowel syndrome, but none of the IBS treatments gave me relief. When it was suggested I might have Crohn's disease, I tried a gluten-free diet. It didn't help. I was treated for bacterial infections and had a full hysterectomy—all in an attempt to alleviate my symptoms. Still, I was stuck with the same problems.

My OB-GYN referred me to a gastroenterologist, and he determined I had a problem with one of my rectal muscles not closing correctly—likely the result of the birth process with one of my children. He thought this might be the reason I didn't have full control over my bowel movements, so I had surgery to correct the problem. It didn't help.

I gave each new health practitioner and each different approach about six months to a year to work before giving up and moving on. I was so frustrated. Sometimes I'd give up for a while and stop seeing any medical practitioners, but I knew I had to find the right care to address my condition. I knew my own body, and I knew what hadn't helped. I started doing my own research, looking for answers.

Eventually, I got to the point where I just learned to live with my condition. If I had to leave the house the next day, I skipped dinner. If I had to travel, I wouldn't eat past lunchtime the day before. I took over-the-counter medication to prevent diarrhea, and I didn't go anywhere unless it was absolutely necessary.

Bowel movements took over my life. There was no way to ignore the fact that an accident could happen at any time. The possibility was very real, and I worried about it constantly. I'd had a few accidents with uncontrolled bowel movements while I was out running errands, and I was highly anxious about it happening again. I couldn't even drive my kids to school in the morning without stopping to use a toilet. I didn't want to embarrass myself, but I also didn't want to embarrass my husband or my kids. I tried to hide my growing anxiety.

Throughout all this, I was still on thyroid medication and still struggling with fatigue, dry skin, and depression. Those were symptoms I could live with—my thyroid symptoms. My intestinal problems, on the other hand, were intolerable. In the end, it was what I had labeled "thyroid symptoms" that ended up leading me to the help I needed with my bowels.

A few of my girlfriends have thyroid problems, and they knew I wasn't well once I stopped going out with them. They kept asking, "How's your thyroid?" I never disclosed my bathroom problems, but I did let them know I was having a hard time balancing my thyroid condition. I told them I'd appreciate any information or ideas they had that might help me.

One day, one of my friends called and I could hear excitement in her voice; she was just bursting with energy and enthusiasm. She'd been sick for some time with a thyroid condition, and I asked her what was going on—why had she called?

She admitted she felt a little guilty that she was feeling so great while some of her friends, like myself, felt lousy. Then she told me she'd been working with a new healthcare provider for a couple of months, and it had completely changed her life. She had been waiting to share this news for some time because she'd wanted to make sure the help she found was the real deal. She didn't want to turn anyone else on to some sort of scam or false promise. But now, she said, it was time.

I was interested, of course, but I was also skeptical. At first I thought: Another diet? Another pill? But as I listened to her story, I began to realize that the type of care she was describing was natural and safe—and clearly, it was working for her. I learned a lot about her thyroid symptoms that day, and it was amazing. I had every single symptom she described!

The practice she recommended wasn't exactly new to me. It was in my local area, and I'd read about it online, but it had never clicked that this practice could really help me. I'd been searching for help for years, and it had been right in front of me. Maybe I just hadn't been quite ready, or maybe I needed "proof" before investing more time, effort, and money into a new health approach. Whatever the reason, it now seemed like it might be the right fit.

I shared everything my friend had said with my husband. The healthcare approach she described involved some pretty radical lifestyle changes and a significant investment, but my husband surprised me by being completely on board with giving it a try. It was then that he finally broke down and told me he was at his wit's end—he wanted our life back as a couple and a family. I called the practice that day.

My husband went with me to my initial consultation, and we could tell right from the start that this practitioner was different. The health practitioner wanted all the details about what I was experiencing and how I coped with it. He was really interested in all of my symptoms, and wanted to know how both my husband and I felt about my health condition and lifestyle. He listened, and when I finally stopped talking, he had a plan.

The first thing he wanted to do was test me for Hashimoto's disease. He told me why he thought I might have it, and explained what it would mean if I did. I learned what was likely causing my body's reaction to food, and what I would probably need to do to heal. Everything he said made sense. I was convinced the lifestyle changes he talked about would help me the way they'd helped my friend, and my husband and I agreed that I needed to get started right away.

As soon as my husband and I walked out of the office and into the parking lot, I burst into tears. I was so relieved! This was the first time a healthcare advisor had given me real hope. I knew it wasn't going to be a quick fix or an easy road to travel, but I didn't care—I would have done anything to get my life back. I was grateful that I'd finally found a way to end my misery.

My test results came back positive for Hashimoto's disease. The care plan my practitioner created for me started with dietary changes and a very specific supplement regimen. I did not eat any gluten, sugar, dairy, salt, or iodine. It was a pretty strict diet by most people's standards, but I didn't care. The first week, I felt better. My bathroom problems were resolved

> # Redd Flag
> Dr. Datis Kharrazian presents some insightful and exciting research on iodine. If you have a primary low thyroid, which is rare in America, iodine can be good for you. But if you have Hashimoto's disease, iodine could be like poison. In fact, iodine could end up being one of the biggest triggers of autoimmune flare-ups.[9(pp. 27-28)]

by about 50%. I didn't have an urgent need to use the toilet after eating, and I wasn't afraid to eat!

A few weeks into my care plan, my husband and I went out to eat together for the first time in years. I made sure we went to restaurants that were willing to help me eat the way I needed to. We definitely had to be a little choosier about where we ate, but that was okay because it was helping. I felt more in control of my body and my life than I had in five years.

The lifestyle changes I made weren't really hard for me, even when results sometimes came slowly. I understood that improvements weren't instantaneous. Eventually, the uncontrollable bowel movements stopped, but I still wasn't "normal." The initial dietary restrictions cleansed my body of toxins so I could have a fresh start, and then we gradually reintroduced foods into my diet one at a time. Some worked for me; others did not.

It turned out that I had a lot of food sensitivities. Until we identified them, I continued to experience some uncomfortable digestive situations. I wasn't instantly healed, but I made progress as the weeks went by. I learned how to notice my body's reactions to what I ate, and how to control any negative reactions. The learning experience was invaluable and is a big part of what allows me to eat with confidence today. I know how to manage my own health, because I know my body.

As time passed, my anxiety faded. I was able to lower the dose of both my thyroid medication and the estrogen I need due to the hysterectomy. My skin looked great; my hair grew in thick and shiny. After about two and half months, I finally shed the baby weight I'd been waiting forever to lose. I lost a total of thirty pounds in four months, and I felt terrific.

I continue to see changes, and I look and feel better every day. The best part is that I'm doing it all through food and nutrition! Today, I'm the one my girlfriends are asking, "What are you doing? You look great and so happy." Now, I don't hesitate to tell everyone I have a thyroid problem, and that I was once very sick. I'm happy to be able to say that I'm managing my health, and these are the results!

My life is different today than it was just a few months ago. For the past four months we've been remodeling our home. Stressful? You bet! But now that I've gained control of my health, I can handle the stress, both physically and mentally. I have the tools I didn't have before—I know what to do.

I wasn't a very fun person to be around for a very long time. I was completely broken. Today, I can travel when I want and be spontaneous without having to worry about being near a bathroom. I go places with my kids and my husband. I relax, have fun, and am able to interact with the world outside my home. It's been worth every ounce of effort, patience, and expense my care plan required. I've regained my personality and my life!

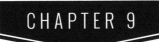

CHAPTER 9

After a Lifetime of Illness, the Future Is Bright

Leslie W.'s Story

The symptoms of Leslie's Hashimoto's disease appeared when she was just a child and played an increasingly detrimental role in her life as she got older. At the height of her illness, Leslie lost more than one successful career and endured the isolation of being bedridden. She was so fatigued that she abandoned her beloved writing and art projects—even reading was too draining.

Once she found the help she needed, Leslie began achieving her dream of wellness so quickly that her current quality of life is nothing short of incredible. Her energy is improved, and she has discovered renewed hope and motivation. Leslie has put those long-abandoned art and writing projects back on her to-do lists, and she's excited about what the future holds.

◇◇◇◇◇◇◇◇◇◇◇◇◇◇◇◇◇◇◇◇◇◇◇◇◇◇◇

"My family—especially my husband, who saw how depressed I was—encouraged me to keep trying to figure out what was going on. I went to [yet] another healthcare advisor who said the same thing: 'There's nothing wrong. Eat less and exercise more.' I tried a third practitioner, who put me on hormone replacement therapy. I was hopeful that this would be the help I desperately needed, but I still felt exhausted and depressed. I didn't lose a pound, and eventually I stopped taking it."

◇◇◇◇◇◇◇◇◇◇◇◇◇◇◇◇◇◇◇◇◇◇◇◇◇◇◇

Ever since I can remember, food has always made me sick. In my family, you finished everything on your plate. I would tell my mother a certain food made me sick, but she'd tell me to eat it anyway because that's all we had.

Most kids look forward to birthday parties and holidays, but I always had some apprehension—I knew it wouldn't be long after the fun started that I'd start feeling ill. It wasn't until I was 12 or 13 that I really started processing what was going on, and wondering why my body reacted to food the way it did.

One of the earliest significant memories I have about health and food happened when I was 13. My grandmother had all of us grandchildren over to her house to help her plan some household jobs. She showed us what needed to be done, and asked which chores we'd like to do next Saturday. Did we want to pull weeds, clean the garage, or paint the fence? Me, I was excited to paint the fence.

The following Saturday was a gorgeous day. My grandmother fed us thick sandwiches, fruit, and homemade cupcakes to give us energy. After lunch, we all went out to begin our chosen chores. After painting just four fence pieces, I had to quit. I felt so tired and lethargic—my arms were like rubber.

My grandmother was angry, and scolded me harshly. She told me how bad I was for being lazy while my cousins were doing all the work. The whole time I was thinking, "Why do I feel so weak? I was fine earlier. What happened? What's wrong with me?" I really wanted to paint the fence for her and to make it look new.

At some point during my teen years, a friend told me that eating wheat makes you fat. I cut it out of my diet immediately, and did lose weight. More importantly, I felt better once I removed wheat from my diet. I didn't know why wheat made me feel sick and tired, but I knew I felt better when I avoided it.

Everyone in my family told me there was no way wheat was making me sick. Even though they said it was all in my head, I was relieved to be feeling a little better.

Once I was in my twenties, I began seeing doctors regularly about my health problems. I knew that if I ate bread or too much sugar I felt nauseous and tired, and I wanted to know why. I was tested for hypoglycemia, but the results showed I was normal. I knew I was really sick, but my practitioners didn't seem to have any answers.

On my own, I continued to identify certain foods that made me feel sick, tired, or suddenly gain weight. I found that the main culprits were grains, sugar, and potatoes. I started making lists of these foods, and stayed away from them as best I could. This helped a little but I was still sick far too often and was lethargic for my age. I knew something other than certain foods was impacting my health—I just didn't know what it was or what to do.

In 1994, my husband and I moved our family to St. George, Utah, and one of the first things we noticed was that people talked a lot about all the local diseases—multiple sclerosis and cancer, for example. After three years in St. George I gained fifty pounds without changing a thing I ate. I tried every diet imaginable and exercised like crazy to try to lose the weight, but nothing helped. I kept gaining. I felt like I had no control over my body, and it was frightening. I started wondering if what we'd heard about the local diseases resulting from atomic bomb fallout could possibly be true; I wondered if I was being affected by radiation.

I eventually gave up on all the diets that didn't work. There was just no point—they all failed. Once I stopped starving myself, I put on 20 more pounds. I was depressed and cried a lot. Finally, my mother suggested I have my thyroid checked, and my grandmother agreed. My husband thought it might be hormonal problems. With so many people pushing me to get checked out, I went to the doctor to have my thyroid and hormone levels tested.

Again, I was told my levels were normal. The practitioner suggested I go on a diet and exercise more. It would be one thing to be told this if I hadn't already tried my hardest to lose weight through diet and exercise, but after all I'd been through I wondered if he just didn't believe me.

My family—especially my husband, who saw how depressed I was—encouraged me to keep trying to figure out what was going on. I went to another healthcare advisor who said the same thing: "There's nothing wrong. Eat less and exercise more." I tried a third practitioner, who put me on hormone replacement therapy. I was hopeful that this would be the help I desperately needed, but I still felt exhausted and depressed. I didn't lose a pound, and eventually I stopped taking it.

For the next 11 years, I cycled through an endless pattern of getting blood tests, hearing I was normal, and seeking help somewhere else. Once we moved to Salt Lake City, I thought I might finally be able to find someone who could figure out what was wrong with me. I saw a new practitioner who told me I had high blood pressure and high cholesterol. I was shocked, because I'd been eating a healthy diet and walking regularly.

I joined a diet program and it took me several months to lose six pounds. But at least it was something. Finally. I was sure this weight-loss program would lower my blood pressure and cholesterol, but when I went back in for testing I learned that those markers had not improved.

This time, I could show my practitioner exactly what I'd been doing with diet and exercise over the past few months on this program. I was prescribed an antidepressant, blood pressure medicine, and more hormone replacement therapy. Not one of these medications helped, and within a few months I'd gained back the six pounds I'd struggled so hard to lose.

My career had always been in business management, and I was an office manager for a long time. As the manager of three departments, I had a busy job. I started hearing people in my office complain that fluorescent lighting could change your heart rhythm and make you feel extra tired. Since I was so exhausted myself, I brought a lamp into my office so I could turn off the overhead fluorescent light; that's how desperate I was to find a solution. My boss thought this was odd, and asked me what was going on. I told him I needed the fluorescent lights turned off because I was fatigued. He just laughed and said, "I think you're nuts."

Ultimately, I ended up leaving my position with that company because I was too worn down to handle the workload. I found a less demanding management position with another company; it was easier work and there wasn't a lot of responsibility. As this new company grew and my duties became more demanding, work became overwhelming again. They kept saying they'd find me an assistant, but it didn't happen quickly enough. I was just too exhausted, and had to resign my position.

Both of these jobs had been excellent careers that I loved. I was sad and confused, and wondered what was happening to me. I found a job as a home health aide assisting elderly clients in their homes. The pay was much lower than what I was accustomed to, but at least I could sit down a lot with this job.

At first, it was easier. Then, the company I worked for started booking me for longer and longer shifts. I told my supervisor she was pushing me too hard, but she said I needed to keep working the long hours. I knew it was going to burn me out, and it did. In 2008, I went into my supervisor's office and actually collapsed in her arms. My mind was as fatigued as my body, and I couldn't think clearly. I didn't know what I was going to do.

My boss put in for a leave of absence for me, and I went home and fell into bed and basically stayed there for the next four and a half years. I just lay there, mostly watching TV. I'm typically a huge reader, but I couldn't read a thing—it was too mentally fatiguing to try to follow more than a few lines at a time.

My social life suffered dramatically. My friends couldn't understand why I didn't want to go out and do things with them anymore. If I tried to talk on the phone for too long, I'd start to fall asleep or lose my train of thought over and over. People would ask me to help with different social luncheons or dinners, and I always had to say no because I just couldn't get up the energy to do anything.

My husband was worried about how fast and how drastically my health had declined. By January 2013, I was completely unable to work outside the home or do chores—even the simplest things were just too taxing.

My husband worked full time and would come home and work, too. He cooked, did all the shopping, cleaned the house, paid the bills, and took care of me. If I was too weak to shower, he would help me. He helped me get dressed. He did everything.

There was a window of just a few minutes every day where I could function—I would get up, get something to eat, take some supplements, go to the bathroom, and then get back in bed. That was my life.

There was a period of about six months where I wanted to end my life. My practitioner wanted to put me on some new medications, but this time I didn't bother. I had no quality of life and I was miserable; I knew pills were not the answer. Only my love for my husband and my kids kept me going.

Over the past 35 years, my family had seen firsthand how certain foods affected me. They would tell me, "Mom, don't eat that—it's going to make you sick." They understood what healthcare professionals seemed unable to explain: my health problems were somehow related to food.

My mother had been what I considered "lazy by choice," but I remember her telling me in the 1960's that she had Hashimoto's disease. I began to rethink her "laziness" once I began experiencing such debilitating symptoms myself. At the same time, I didn't want to be like my mother! I had things I wanted to do. I loved to write, and there were three different books I had intended to complete. I loved painting, but I hadn't been able to paint in years. I was weak, I had the shakes, and I couldn't do much of anything. Sometimes I had the drive to complete projects or chores, but my body was like a ball and chain dragging me down.

I had one girlfriend who was very compassionate. When I would feel good, which happened about once every three months, I would get dressed and go see her for an hour or two. Then I'd turn around and come home and that would be my one outing for the next few months.

It's hard for people to understand how sick you are when you have no diagnosis. I'd fix myself up, dress nice, go out, and people would think I was fine. Then, when I told them I had to pace myself and be careful with my energy, they'd look at me like I was crazy. They didn't understand that I couldn't just sit down and regain strength; it would take me days or weeks to recoup even the smallest amount of energy.

I desperately wanted a better quality of life, and I had plenty of time to think about how much better things could be. I never really stopped looking for help. It's ironic that being practically bedridden is the reason I found what I was looking for.

One day I saw a health practitioner talking about low thyroid symptoms on TV. I had every symptom. I figured this man had to know what he was talking about if he could string together every single one of my symptoms. He also appeared to understand what might be causing them. Even so, I was skeptical.

I did some research and discovered that this practitioner had a good reputation for helping low thyroid and Hashimoto's patients. The more I read and learned about him, the more I was convinced that this was what I needed. I booked an appointment with an endocrinologist and had her do some extensive blood work, which showed that I did have Hashimoto's disease.

The following week, I went for a consultation with the practitioner I'd seen on TV. I dragged myself in there along with all of my blood work—the current tests, plus all the ones I'd had done for the past ten years. You can imagine my surprise when, after seeing all that, he wanted to do more tests of his own.

After looking at all of my results, he explained in detail what was happening in my body. I wasn't prepared to hear how seriously ill I was, even though I knew how bad I felt. Deep down, I was still hoping for a simple answer. I received completely new information about how my body was suffering with inflammation due to the autoimmune disease.

The most frightening thing I learned was that if I didn't get my condition under control, it would get worse.

At the end of my visit, I realized it was within my power to get well and stay well. I wanted to control my disease because I wanted quality of life; ultimately, it really was that simple. I made a commitment to get on this practitioner's program and follow the protocol he designed for me.

My care plan started out with a very specific diet and nutritional supplements to calm my immune system. Even though it was restrictive, it wasn't hard to do. Each day I felt better, and I was motivated by how quickly my health turned around. Within the first month, my blood pressure was normal. At my three-month mark, I'd lost 21 pounds and my cholesterol was much lower. I continued to lose an average of two pounds a week, and I never had to count calories or measure food. In fact, I ate as much as I wanted spread out in several small meals each day. I ate according to what my body could tolerate and

Redd Flag

Leslie was suffering with Hashimoto's autoimmune reaction. This means her immune system was attacking her thyroid and she had symptoms of Hashimoto's, but she did not yet have a permanent low thyroid.[24, 25] Leslie's TSH markers were all within normal range, so she did not require thyroid medication.

Healthcare practitioners often monitor the progression of this condition and start treatment only when the thyroid no longer produces hormones efficiently.[9(pp. 24-25)] This delayed treatment can be frustrating for patients who are experiencing debilitating symptoms despite having lab results in the normal range.

In fact, this period before permanent low thyroid occurs is the most optimal time to help patients with Hashimoto's. Identifying and managing the physiological, dietary, and lifestyle factors that trigger the patient's autoimmune reaction can make a dramatic impact on the patient's future and quality of life.

followed the protocol.

Four months after I started my care plan, I was having more and more good days and had lost a total of 34 pounds. I was thrilled! My practitioner was confident that my health and energy would continue to improve, and it did.

Today, I am as active as ever and feel completely "normal" most of the time—I feel like myself. I've regained my drive and am starting to accomplish the goals I had to put on hold. My shakes are gone, and I have been able to start painting again. I still have unexplained down days every once in awhile, but nothing nearly as bad as what I lived with in the past.

Life has brought me unexpected challenges over the past year, and my improved health has allowed me to bounce back from the hard times. I recently lost my companion pet of 17 years at the same time I was struggling with other emotionally difficult circumstances, and I was absolutely devastated. Although the loss flattened me, I was able to recover by using the knowledge I'd gained about caring for my health.

Despite these challenges, this year also brought various achievements and tremendous joy. There were a few weeks when my son needed help with his business, and I had enough energy to help him for a couple hours every day.

Perhaps the most tremendous testament to my health is that I took in a foster child about a year ago. I have always wanted to foster a teenage daughter, and I was finally healthy enough to do it. We do a lot of fun things together, and she runs circles around me! I would never have had the energy to foster a teenage daughter or help my son with his work if it wasn't for my practitioner and his clinic. I'm doing more now than I have in nearly a decade, and I owe him everything.

During the four and a half years I was home sick in bed, my pets and my family gave me unconditional love—I knew I mattered, and that was a big part of what kept me going. Now, I have a lifestyle I can maintain that will keep me healthy. When I see the quote that says "Live, Love,

Laugh," I can finally relate! In the years to come, I'll be traveling and enjoying my family, and spending my energy serving others in ways I enjoy. I'm looking forward to a lifetime of love and adventures.

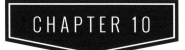
Thyroid Problems Can and Do Affect Men

Aaron's Story

Aaron's story reveals two surprising but important facts about thyroid conditions: intense, debilitating symptoms can impact even a young, healthy man, and those symptoms can appear in body systems that may seem completely unrelated to the thyroid.

As a husband, father of three, and very active man in his mid-thirties, Aaron had always thrived in a fast-paced lifestyle. Then, in 2011, he became so sick within the span of a week that it was impossible for him to even climb stairs. Aaron's symptoms of uncontrolled Hashimoto's disease were so severe that he found himself face-to-face with a cardiologist who told him he needed major heart surgery.

◇◇◇◇◇◇◇◇◇◇◇◇◇◇◇◇◇◇◇◇◇◇◇◇◇◇◇◇

"My wife would ask me what was wrong but I couldn't tell her because I really didn't know. That was a huge source of frustration, too—the not knowing. The only thing I knew was that I felt so bad I wanted to die. Absolutely nothing sounded good or enjoyable to me."

◇◇◇◇◇◇◇◇◇◇◇◇◇◇◇◇◇◇◇◇◇◇◇◇◇◇◇◇

I'm typically a very active guy. I always spent my free time participating in outdoor activities with my family or working on some project around the house. At the end of the day, I slept great because I was tired in a good, natural way. Combined with my age and the fact that I had always felt fine, it was shocking when I started having major health problems. The first indication something was wrong with my health were symptoms that appeared to be heart-related.

It was Christmas break when I first noticed my heart rate was irregular. I could actually feel my heart racing, especially at night—it was so intense that it interfered with my sleep. I checked my pulse and blood pressure, and what I discovered was pretty alarming: my pulse was around 110 to 120, and my blood pressure was 160/120.

A day or two later I started feeling constantly uncomfortable, even just sitting on the couch. My circulatory system was pounding, and nothing I did seemed to calm it down. At almost the exact same time, my energy plummeted. I had no energy; even lifting my arms or legs to get up and walk across the room was exhausting. I'm 6' 8," and at the time I was 285 pounds. Although 33 seemed a little young for heart problems, I went to see a cardiologist because I was worried about my blood pressure and my extreme fatigue.

The cardiologist did an EKG and said he could understand why I was feeling so awful—my blood pressure and pulse were very high. He immediately started talking about surgery, and how he could go through an artery in my thigh to access parts of my heart that were misfiring. I remember just sitting there in the exam room in a state of shock, wondering if I was hearing him wrong. Just a week before, I'd felt fine! I made him repeat himself a few times,

Redd Flag

Many low thyroid patients have had heart palpitations or a racing heart so severe that it felt as if they may be having a heart attack. This is because as the immune system destroys the thyroid, it releases a large amount of thyroid hormones into the blood stream. This causes hyperthyroid symptoms, such as heart palpitations.

People suffering with Hashimoto's have the worst of both worlds. They may have all of the low thyroid symptoms, plus all of the hyperthyroid symptoms while their condition is flared.[20]

just to be sure I'd understood correctly. When it became clear that this wasn't just some big misunderstanding, I practically flew out of my seat to get to the door. I muttered something about needing a second opinion, and told him I wasn't ready for surgery. I wanted some evidence to show there was really something that serious going on.

Although he was still gung ho about surgery, he did calm me down and get me seated again. Then, he asked about my thyroid. I said I'd never had thyroid problems that I knew of, but my parents and my sister had been on thyroid medication for most of their lives. That bit of information seemed to point him in a different direction, and he decided to refer me to an endocrinologist. I left the cardiologist's office with a glimmer of hope that I might avoid a surgical procedure; I was relieved to learn I might not have heart disease.

This health crisis gave me a pretty good scare, and I began to really watch what I ate. I'd started exercising as soon as I saw the cardiologist, even though it was still a massive struggle to move at all. I was exhausted, but I forced myself to do it. I kept thinking about my wife and my

> ## Redd Flag
> Imagine if Aaron had gone through with heart surgery when his problems had nothing to do with the heart—his "heart symptoms" were caused by an overproduction of thyroid hormones.

kids and how awful it would be if something really major happened to me. Despite how hard I pushed and how careful I was with what I ate, my weight climbed.

I went up to 294 pounds. I'd never been that heavy in my life, and it only added to my exhaustion. Still, nothing I did seemed to help me lose any weight. In the past, if I put on a few pounds over the holidays, all it took was a little extra activity to drop them. This time, I just kept gaining. I barely ate anything but I still kept putting on the pounds.

When I went in to see the endocrinologist, he ordered blood work and started working on a diagnosis right away. He determined that I had a thyroid problem, and started me on thyroid medication.

Unfortunately, the medicine didn't do a thing to make me feel better, and I actually started to feel worse the longer I was on it. I experienced uncomfortable side effects: I started breaking out in hives and rashes, and I had headaches. At least three times a week, I'd end up with a migraine that lasted all day. I still couldn't sleep, and I had to push myself just to stay awake long enough to get through the workday. I dreaded waking up. I no longer found any joy in life. My job seemed too demanding— even just driving there and home again was taxing.

I ended up seeing three different endocrinologists over the course of that year, hoping to find a medication that would work or a dosage that would help me. I spent a ton of time on healthcare visits and lab work, and a lot of hard-earned cash on copayments for visits and medications. It was money we really could have used for other things. Every time I filled another prescription, I grew more and more frustrated at the lack of results.

I eventually realized all the healthcare professionals seemed to have the same goal: correct my TSH levels. I didn't feel like they were really concerned about how I felt, or that they cared what was causing the problem in the first

Redd Flag

Earlier, we learned that Hashimoto's patients can exercise intensely and maintain a strict diet and still gain weight if nothing is being done to correct the root cause of the problem.[9(pp. 27-28)] In patients with Hashimoto's, an enzyme called hormone-sensitive lipase (HSL), which helps break down fat,[26] may shut down.

Additionally, many patients have significant metabolic imbalances that prevent the breakdown of fat and encourage the body to store glucose as fat.

Unfortunately, family, friends, and others may incorrectly assume that these patients are simply lazy and eat too much. These assumptions couldn't be further from the truth, and can be detrimental to the patient's state of mind and to their physical health.

place. They also didn't seem concerned about all the time and money I was spending on "fixes" that failed.

As awful as I felt and as frustrated as I was, it was nothing compared to how bad I felt for my family. I wasn't a very good dad during this time. My kids were 11, 9, and 4 years old, and they really didn't understand how sick I was; all they knew was that I couldn't play with them or take them places, and I was often short-tempered. The only thing I really wanted in the evenings was to be left alone so I could try to rest and get up enough strength to work the next day. Even today, my heart hurts just thinking about what my health problems caused me to put my kids through.

I wasn't a great husband, either. I was a bump on a log. When it was obvious I was frustrated, my wife would ask me what was wrong but I couldn't tell her because I really didn't know. That was a huge source of frustration, too—the not knowing. The only thing I knew was that I felt so bad I wanted to die. Absolutely nothing sounded good or enjoyable to me.

Everyone who talked to me annoyed me. I wasn't a very nice person to my wife or my co-workers, and I wasn't kind to people I met day-to-day, like in shops. This was completely unlike how I used to be, and I couldn't stand myself. I had no idea how to get back to the person I used to be. It was like someone had pulled the cord on my life and I couldn't figure out how to plug it back in.

Things finally began to change when I started talking to a health practitioner I knew from church. I'd been doing some research online for thyroid help in my area, and came across his website. The next time I saw him, I approached him. He asked me a few questions and I could tell he was completely unlike any other healthcare professional I'd seen. He seemed to understand what my symptoms meant and what they were all adding up to.

I made an appointment at his practice and went in to see him shortly after our first conversation. He reviewed the blood work he had ordered, and I'll never forget what he said: "You have Hashimoto's disease. You're also pre-diabetic, your blood pressure and cholesterol are elevated, your liver enzymes and inflammatory markers are high, and you're extremely dehydrated." Great news, right? Well, to me it actually was! I knew how I felt, and he knew how sick I really was. I was sure he had the map that could get me back on the path to my former life. I jumped on board with his plan and didn't get off until I hit my goal, which was the way the "old me" had felt at a weight of 230 pounds.

I started working with this practitioner in October. Over the next five months, I dropped 69 pounds just by changing what I ate and taking nutritional supplements. It's still amazing to me that this involved no exercise and no weight loss program. I didn't have to starve myself; it was simply a matter of eating in a way that allowed my body to heal.

My diet focused on vegetables, fruits, chicken, and natural grains. No dairy and no gluten. Within the first week, I started feeling better. I felt lighter in a way that went beyond weight loss—my body stopped feeling weighed down and bloated.

I'm now off all medication, including blood pressure and thyroid pills. I'm healthy again, and I didn't need surgery or a ton of medication to get back to feeling great. I feel like I did when I was a senior in high school. I have so much energy! Running is easier, being a dad is easier—even working is easier. Before I started healing, I could barely stay awake at work despite consuming tons of caffeine. Now my body is functioning as it should and I don't even think about caffeine. I sleep great, I have a great outlook on life, and I'm back to being my old self. I can enjoy my family again, and they can enjoy me.

People don't believe me when I tell them I really didn't exercise. In fact, a big part of my healing was giving my body a chance to rest. All the exercise I'd done—all the dieting—really wasn't helping. In fact, it was making me worse. I gradually became more active as I felt better, but there was no struggle at all to lose weight once my liver started functioning and I was no longer dehydrated.

I still don't eat dairy; I use almond milk instead. If I accidentally eat something with gluten, I can tell within about three hours. My wife can tell, too. She knows if I'm short tempered, it's probably something I ate. We go over what I had and can usually pinpoint the culprit. She's not afraid to ask me if I've gotten sloppy about my diet! It's actually a help to me, and we're both relieved about that. We have answers now, and we can talk about my health problems in a way that can make things better.

I do my own cooking most of the time, but my wife does her best to keep plenty of gluten-free foods in the house. She supports me completely, and so do my kids. They understand that as long as I watch what I eat, for the most part, I feel good.

There's maybe a day or two out of the month where I have a lapse or don't feel so great, but that's something my practitioner has said is pretty normal. There is no cure for Hashimoto's, but, if you can identify your triggers, you can get to a point where about 25 days out of the month are good ones. For anyone with Hashimoto's, feeling great is totally doable once you're shown the way.

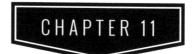
Not Your Typical Thyroid Symptoms

Seth's Story

Most healthcare providers associate low thyroid conditions with women—specifically, women who are 40 or older. Seth's case is an exception; not only is he male, but his health problems began in his mid-20s. To compound the uncharacteristic nature of his illness, Seth experienced symptoms that are not typically associated with thyroid disorders. The uncommon nature of his illness made it difficult for him to find the help he needed to regain his health.

Seth's story is just one example of why we don't rule out Hashimoto's disease simply because gender, age, or symptoms are atypical of the illness. If you're experiencing symptoms of a thyroid disorder, or are suffering from unexplained symptoms, you may have an undiagnosed autoimmune disease of the thyroid. There is hope, and there is help.

◇◇◇◇◇◇◇◇◇◇◇◇◇◇◇◇◇◇◇◇◇◇

"Some days, I could barely pull myself out of bed in the morning.
Who wants to face the day when you're uncomfortable, exhausted,
and in so much pain you can barely stand?"

◇◇◇◇◇◇◇◇◇◇◇◇◇◇◇◇◇◇◇◇◇◇

My health problems first began about five years ago. I was newly married, and my wife and I were living in married student housing at Utah State University in Logan, Utah. I was going to school and working, and we were both focused and excited about the future. One day, I woke up with a rash covering almost my entire body. I had red splotches and bumps from head to toe, and I itched so badly it was almost unbearable.

I'd always been healthy and physically fit, and I never had any allergies, so my wife and I were shocked at the sudden appearance of the rash. We had no idea what could possibly be causing it. I hadn't done anything unusual in the previous days; there had been no apparent changes in my diet, at our apartment, or in my surroundings. All we could think was that maybe some sort of insect bit me, or that I had somehow been exposed to a harsh chemical that caused an allergic reaction.

I went to the doctor immediately to have it checked out, thinking I'd probably need some sort of antihistamine or cream prescription. He recommended oatmeal baths, avoiding hot showers, and using over the counter cortisol creams. Nothing seemed to help, so he referred me to someone else. He was the first in a long line of practitioners I cycled through in the area: allergy specialists, dermatologists, and various other practitioners. None of them could figure out what was going on.

Despite the fact that I was swollen, constantly itching, and in a good amount of pain, I finished my semester and we moved to Salt Lake City so I could start a new job. I figured I'd start seeing practitioners in Salt Lake City about my rash as soon as possible, but once we arrived the rash disappeared as quickly as it had started.

Since nobody had been able to figure out what caused the rash, my wife and I began to think that maybe there was some mold in the old building where we'd been living—maybe that was what I'd reacted to. Whatever the cause, I was thankful and relieved that the rash was gone. We lived in Salt Lake City for 16 months, and I never had any sign of a rash the entire time. After a while, I forgot about it.

Unfortunately, things weren't just that easy.

My wife and I moved to Provo, Utah so I could return to school and attend the police academy. We were back in student housing, and I'd secured arrangements to work as a night watchman at the residence.

It allowed us to get a good discount on our apartment, which made it more affordable to live there. It also freed me up to go to classes during the day and attend the academy in the evenings. It was the ideal setup to allow me to work as efficiently as possible toward my goals.

After only a couple of weeks in our new apartment, signs of the rash returned. It was the beginning of another health nightmare; the rash came back full force. I lived with it every single day for over a year. I was miserable.

This wasn't like a rash that was just sort of "there." It itched horribly, nonstop, and if I scratched it, it spread. Hot water made it worse, so I started taking cold showers. My wife and I tried again and again to figure out what could be triggering it. We changed detergents and soaps, and kept checking for some kind of bug that could be biting me. I started seeing specialists again. Nothing helped.

Living with this condition was like having some sort of awful monster constantly attacking me. I could never get it to calm down enough for me to feel normal, although cooler temperatures kept it from raging. The warm summer months were the worst.

If I worked out and started sweating, the rash spread like crazy. The pain and itching nearly drove me mad. We tried every kind of rash cream, prescription, and home

Redd Flag

Seth is suffering with chronic idiopathic urticaria (CIU)—long-lasting hives of unknown origin.[27] Recent research shows that most CIU patients have what is called chronic autoimmune urticaria.[28] Steroids and antihistamines provide little to no improvement for chronic autoimmune urticaria because the condition is caused by the immune system turning on itself.

Remember: when you have one autoimmune disease, you're likely to have other autoimmune diseases as well. Clinically, we see a strong correlation between CIU and autoimmune low thyroid, and research supports this association.[29] Tempering the inflammatory process as swiftly as possible tends to quickly reduce or even eliminate the hives.

remedy you can name. Nothing worked. In time, I began to think this was something I'd just have to deal with for the rest of my life.

My classmates at the police academy were worried about me. Classes were mandatory, so I had to be there every day. If my classmates hadn't been there to support me, I would probably have skipped classes and failed the academy. Some days I was covered in red spots; other days my face and lips were so swollen and puffy that I didn't even look like me. Every day I'd hear, "What's wrong with you?" I'd say I had allergies, but I really had no idea what was going on. I felt like I had no control over my own body. It was terrifying.

After seeing who knows how many practitioners, I finally met with one who ran some in-depth tests and told me I had Hashimoto's disease. At the time, the only thing this meant to me was that I had to start taking thyroid medication.

I was still seeing other practitioners to try to figure out my rash, even though I had virtually no faith they could help me. I was desperate for relief. I saw at least six different medical professionals over 18 months, including family practice physicians, dermatologists, an

> ## Redd Flag
> Seth's immune system was attacking multiple parts of his body. The amount of inflammation caused significant problems. In a situation like Seth's, a lack of proper care can compound the existing problems.

ear, nose and throat doctor, two endocrinologists, and another allergy specialist. I still couldn't get rid of the rash.

I couldn't sleep because I was constantly itching and feeling hot and in pain. I was exhausted all the time from lack of sleep and from physically and mentally fighting this rash. I started suffering from really bad joint pain, too. I was 26 years old—way too young for arthritis! Some days, I could barely pull myself out of bed in the morning. Who wants to face the day when you're uncomfortable, exhausted, and in so much pain you can barely stand?

I've always considered myself to be an athlete—someone in good physical shape—but the training at the police academy was incredibly hard for me. Physical activities that would have been easy just a few months before were barely manageable. I understood the academy wasn't supposed to be "easy," but I was really struggling. Running was especially difficult because I had so much pain in my knees. I'd hoped to really excel at the academy. Instead, I just barely squeaked by.

I was under constant stress knowing everyone could see that there was something physically wrong with me. I was embarrassed to leave the house because my face would get so disfigured from the swelling. It was one of the most difficult times of my life.

Eventually, I began to notice that certain foods seemed to make things worse. Dairy products would make the rash flare up more severely, so I started staying away from them. I now know that I had a lot more food sensitivities going on than I could have ever figured out on my own. At the time, I was so desperate to feel better that just a tiny bit of relief from avoiding dairy felt like a huge success.

I started studying allergies and Hashimoto's disease. I researched in books and online. I knew it was up to me to find the help I needed. Finally, late last summer, I found a wellness center that looked promising.

The first thing that caught

Redd Flag

It's incredible that one simple trigger can flare up autoimmunity, creating a huge mess within the body.[30] Avoiding dietary triggers can make a tremendous difference.

Understanding that you don't feel bad without reason is significant. If you feel more inflamed or feel your symptoms return or worsen, ask yourself, "What did I do differently?" There is always something that is causing a flare up, and it's up to you to be the detective and determine what it is. If you can't do it on your own, enlist the support of a healthcare practitioner. Functional medicine or personalized lifestyle medicine practices or clinics may be able to help.

my eye about this practice was their approach. I was watching the practitioner's videos on YouTube, and he stressed again and again that it was possible to heal from the inside out. I was already aware that what I ate sometimes made the rash worse, and the idea of healing through diet caught my attention. Creams and potions and pills certainly hadn't helped.

I felt incredibly lucky that this practitioner was fairly local to my area. I told my wife I wanted to schedule a consultation, and she told me to go for it. She wanted me well again, and she'd also started to suspect—even more strongly than I did—that this rash had something to do with food and nutrition.

Naturally, we were both skeptical after all the trials and failures of so many healthcare practitioners. After my first consultation, I knew right away that this was the program that could help me. The practitioner wasn't baffled or even overly surprised at my symptoms—not even the rash! He said he'd seen cases like mine before. He knew right away what was happening to me, and he was confident he'd be able to help me.

The practitioner's care plan was much more involved than just "watching my diet." It was a systematic approach to getting my body's inflammation under control. I had to heal my leaky gut so my foods could nourish me and I could regain my energy. The focus was on healing from the inside out through a careful diet and specific supplements. Once my body was functioning better, we added foods back into my diet to learn what I can and can't tolerate.

My wife was thrilled to hear that my practitioner was recommending a major lifestyle change. At the time, my schedule was terrible. I had school during the day, and then I attended the police academy in the evenings.

> ## Redd Flag
> One lifestyle factor that often requires modification for autoimmune patients is sleep patterns. Working night shifts can contribute to elevated and fluctuating cortisol levels,[31] which can exacerbate autoimmunity.[32]

At night, I worked as a watchman at our apartment's property. It was just crazy, the hours I was trying to keep.

I'm convinced that my schedule was a major contributing factor, if not the number one cause, of a lot of my health problems. My wife hated seeing me so sick and unhappy, and she had already realized that my schedule needed to change if I was going to get better. When my health practitioner said I really needed a normal schedule and more regular hours to help my body heal, she was all over making it happen. She was the major driving force in getting us moved back to Salt Lake City.

Within the first week on my diet, which was designed to calm down my body's inflammation, the rash started going away! It's hard to explain how it felt to experience such quick relief with just dietary changes. Once the rash retreated, it was easy to stay on track with what was a pretty restrictive diet. I say "retreated," because it felt like something I'd been battling every day for over a year. I was telling everyone, "Look, I don't have a rash anymore!" My energy started to climb that first week, too. I could exercise without excruciating pain. In no time, it felt good to be moving my body and I started to enjoy working out again.

When I started getting such great results, my first thought was that I must be allergic to a whole bunch of different foods. My practitioner said this wasn't likely and that once my body was healthy again, I'd be able to eat more foods—we'd introduce them slowly. He was right. There are certain foods I still need to avoid due to sensitivities, but my diet is by no means as restrictive as it was when I first started my care plan.

My practitioner had the knowledge and experience to help me through the healing process, and he gave me the education I would need to take care of my health long-term. There is just no way I would ever have been able to do it on my own; I think it was one of the best decisions we ever made.

I've come a long way since my doctor first saw me last year. My wife and I have put down some roots and slowed the pace of our lives. We recently bought our first home and we've been living in it for about three weeks now. I graduated from the police academy and am on the waiting list for an officer's job. In the meantime, I'm working in retail. Since we moved to Salt Lake City, I no longer have to deal with night watchman hours. I'm awake when other people are awake, and I get enough sleep most of the time.

I've also completely changed my diet. I have time to eat properly now, and I invest the effort required to live a healthier, calmer life. Sometimes I still have trouble falling asleep, but it's nothing like the way I used to struggle. I'm still learning how to keep a good, regular schedule. Major life changes don't happen overnight; I understand it's a process, and I'm comfortable with that.

I haven't seen any sign of the rash since last fall. Some days I don't have much energy, or I may have some aches and pains, but I'm confident I'm well on my way to getting my energy back to the level it once was. I can go for a run and barely break a sweat. I don't have any problems with

> ## Redd Flag
>
> We have found that when autoimmunity is flared, the patient is intolerant to many more foods than when things are calmed down. It's important to identify what foods you have to avoid when things are calmed down and what foods you have to avoid when you are in a major flare up. They may be quite different.

puffiness or swelling in my face. Let me say it again: the rash is gone! Not only that, but I know it's not coming back. I'm finally in control of my health.

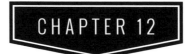

CHAPTER 12

Unable to Even Get Out of Bed

Heather's Story

Heather loves her life as a successful artist and wife. Her busy, creative lifestyle and career demand a lot of energy, and her upbeat outlook and enthusiasm for life are a big part of her personality.

Heather once suffered with such severe thyroid symptoms that she struggled to get out of bed each morning. She was able to overcome serious obstacles and regain her health by relying on the one thing she knew she had: belief in herself and the power of autonomy.

◇◇◇◇◇◇◇◇◇◇◇◇◇◇◇◇◇◇◇◇◇◇◇◇◇◇

"I had no motivation to work and no energy to spend time with my husband. I'd always been thin; now I was chunky and still gaining weight. My husband was worried at first, but after a while I knew he was also getting frustrated. Sometimes I'd catch a look that just felt like he was thinking, 'Who on earth did I marry?'"

◇◇◇◇◇◇◇◇◇◇◇◇◇◇◇◇◇◇◇◇◇◇◇◇◇◇

Today, I'm a lot like I was when I was young—really energetic and always in a good mood! I was a thin, athletic girl, and I loved participating in sports and staying busy. It wasn't until I was about 20 that I first started struggling with health problems. When those problems hit, they hit hard; it was as if my entire personality changed and the creative energy that drives me grinded to a halt.

I went to see my doctor because I was living in a chronic state of exhaustion. I was completely worn out and exhausted, but when bedtime finally arrived I couldn't fall asleep. My mind wanted to rest and I was so physically tired that I could barely move, but sleep just wouldn't come. I'd feel even worse the next day—it was a horrible cycle. My doctor tested my thyroid and told me I was hypothyroid. Then he ran some more tests and diagnosed me with Hashimoto's disease.

I took these diagnoses at face value and listened to what my healthcare provider said: he told me I'd need to take medication every day for the rest of my life. I wanted to feel better, so I took the medication. The problem was, the medication didn't work. I kept waiting for the night I'd crawl into bed and drift off to sleep like I always used to—like a normal person—but that never happened.

At the time, I was fresh out of college where I'd studied graphic design; I was a newlywed, eager to start a career and enjoy my new life with my husband. As time passed, I started to feel even worse. I became depressed, and gained fifteen pounds in less than three months. At that point, things really began to go downhill; what had started out bad turned into a complete nightmare. My life came to a halt. I had no motivation to work and no energy to spend time with my husband. I'd always been thin; now I was chunky and still gaining weight. My husband was worried at first, but after a while I knew he was also getting frustrated. Sometimes I'd catch a look that just felt like he was thinking, "Who on earth did I marry?"

I knew what was happening to my health wasn't right, so I went back to my practitioner and told him how horrible I was feeling. He said my thyroid dose wasn't right, and that he'd adjust it. In my mind, that made absolutely no sense—I should feel at least a little bit better on thyroid medication, even if the dose is too low.

I started doing research on Hashimoto's disease and low thyroid, and what I learned was pretty shocking. I realized that what was going on in my body was much more complicated than I'd imagined, and that my condition would be difficult to regulate. I also learned that a simple fix wasn't likely to help me feel good. The good news was, I felt like my experience was validated in some way. I wasn't just crazy!

I started seeing different health practitioners at that point. I wanted my life back, and I didn't give up. I knew the thyroid medicine wasn't working, and I knew I wasn't eating too much. I finally found a general practitioner who was willing to switch me to a natural thyroid replacement, and I started to feel a little better. My fatigue wasn't as extreme on this medication, but I definitely still didn't feel like myself.

I spent the next five years in that state of limbo. Looking back, I don't know how my marriage survived. I took the medication and did what I could to eat healthy and exercise, but I felt awful. I'm naturally a happy, excited, and motivated person; I'm creative and ambitious, and I always have a lot of projects I'm working on or planning. During those years, though, I didn't want to do anything. I didn't care about anything. Honestly, I just wanted to sleep and be left alone.

The way I was feeling was the opposite of how I used to feel, and it was so depressing. I knew I wasn't making the most of my life—not even close! I watched the years go by: 23, 24, 25. I lived like a very old, sick person instead of a young woman who should be out having fun.

My libido was low, and this caused some heartbreaking issues in my marriage. I didn't feel like being romantic with my husband—I rejected him, and in time he stopped trying. I felt completely unattractive and was in a lot of pain, both physically and emotionally. My hair was falling out. I was overweight. My joints hurt constantly, and my bones felt like they were burning and aching all the time. I developed bursitis in my hips. Every morning I'd wake up and cry because I didn't want to get out of bed. It hurt too much, and I felt I had nothing to look forward to—nothing to live for.

Still, I kept researching my condition. Celiac disease, another autoimmune disease, kept coming up in connection with Hashimoto's.

I learned that it's common to have multiple autoimmune diseases, and I began to realize I needed to focus on much more than my thyroid.

I ended up back at a practitioner's office with this new information in hand. When it turned out I did have Celiac disease, the doctor told me, "You need to cut out gluten." It may sound simple, but there was really nothing simple about it. I was an avid baker; cutting out gluten was a very big deal for me.

But, I was determined to get better so I focused on learning how to remove gluten from my

Redd Flag

Maintaining a gluten-free diet can be a daunting task, and it's not as simple as avoiding products that contain wheat, barley and rye. There are so many different products and ingredients that contain gluten. For example, malt from barley and bulgur (which is a form of wheat) contains gluten. Even modified starches can contain gluten.[33,34]

diet. It wasn't easy, but it was worth the effort because I did see quite a bit of improvement. The swelling went down in my face, and I didn't feel quite as tired. There was a real difference in how I looked and felt; it was encouraging.

I was learning that it was possible to take care of myself and manage my Celiac disease by modifying my diet. I didn't feel great, but I was happy to feel even a little bit better. I believed the pain and extra weight and tiredness were things I'd just have to deal with for the rest of my life. My thyroid problem and the Hashimoto's disease loomed over my head, but there didn't seem to be anything I could do about it.

At that point, I'd gone as far as I could on my own. Just when I needed it, help came my way. My sister told me about someone she knew who had autoimmune diseases. This person had gone to a clinic and achieved remarkable results through diet and supplementation.

Hearing this person's success story really motivated me. The fact that the program was completely different—an alternative approach that actually helped someone—made me excited. In the back of my mind I felt like this was what I'd been waiting for, and I wanted to experience the same amazing results myself.

I made an appointment for a consultation at the practice my sister's friend recommended. When I went in, it was like stepping into a different world—a world where my condition wasn't a big mystery. This place helped people like me all the time!

My new healthcare practitioner ran tests that were far more in depth and detailed than anything I'd ever seen or heard of before. When the results were in, my husband came with me to review the findings. The practitioner explained everything that was malfunctioning in my body. As terrible as I felt, I was appalled to learn just how poorly my body was really functioning. It was a very difficult appointment to sit through.

The tests showed that my liver wasn't functioning well and my adrenal glands were completely out of whack. My hormones were imbalanced, and I had leaky gut syndrome. I was vitamin D deficient, too, among other things.

After the appointment, I got in the car with my husband and cried for about ten minutes. It was terrifying to learn all the details about my illnesses. I knew autoimmune conditions were complicated, but I was in no way prepared for the level and extent of dysfunction those tests revealed.

I was also overwhelmed thinking about how much work this program was going to be. All the responsibility would be on me—they weren't going to just hand me a pill and say, "You'll get better now." I would need to make a huge commitment: appointments twice a week and following a strict diet.

I knew it was going to be a process that would require time and dedication, but I realized that this was really what I'd searched for all along. Ultimately, it was up to me to change my eating habits and do whatever it would take to make myself better; I'd learned a long time ago that no healthcare professional could do this for me. I started to imagine what it would be like six months down the road, and I got really excited! I felt better already.

I started this program about two weeks after hearing my lab results. Each time I had an appointment, the practitioner explained to me exactly what I needed to be doing and why. Every step of the way, he explained the science that supported his recommendations. I loved that! It wasn't just someone telling me what to do; instead, I was learning why I was doing what I was doing so I could understand my body processes. Everything was based on recent research in top medical journals. It was a systematic approach—there were no theories or guesswork involved.

For me, the first step was taking supplements to help improve my most significant imbalances. I also removed all inflammatory foods for a month or so. In just those first few weeks, I noticed a huge difference in my body. The painful bursitis I had in my hips vanished. I went from taking tons of ibuprofen to taking absolutely nothing at all. My husband and I had been considering moving to a home without stairs because I had such difficulty getting around, but my joints started feeling so much better that we no longer needed to think about leaving our home. The pain had disappeared!

I noticed a huge difference in my energy levels, too. That first week I was really tired because I wasn't having any caffeine, but by the second week I was sleeping better and had more energy. My mood improved dramatically. I felt so much more like myself—I hadn't felt that way in years.

At that point I knew what I was doing was working. I continued with the supplements and elimination diet, and felt better and better. Then, my practitioner started adding foods back in one at a time. It was an eye-opening, amazing experience. If I felt unwell when we'd add a food back in, then I knew it was something I would need to eliminate long term. I discovered that I could know within a few hours if a food was triggering for me or not; I could literally feel the difference once I learned how to pay attention.

Any time I had questions I contacted my healthcare provider, and the practitioner or a member of his support staff would call me right back. I was never rushed off the phone. If I felt different one week or was not doing so great, I explained what was going on and they would adjust things accordingly. I'd tried going gluten-free alone, and struggled with it, so I appreciated this clinic's attentive approach so much. It made a world of difference for me.

I continued with the program and kept feeling better and better. Four months after I started, we ran a second round of lab work to evaluate my progress. I was expecting to see a little bit of improvement, but I was completely blown away by the results. Everything had made a complete 180. My thyroid test results were much improved, and I'd stopped taking thyroid medication at the beginning of the program so the improvements had nothing to do with pills. My adrenal function completely turned around. My liver was functioning well, and my vitamin D levels were better.

The way my body was functioning had completely changed. I knew then that if I ever had health problems going forward, I could bounce back. I could take care of myself through diet and supplements, and could manage my thyroid without medication.

It's incredible how different my life is now. Not long ago, my husband lost his job and I took on a really stressful position to increase our income. There is no way I would have been able to handle this before. The extra money I made ultimately allowed me to quit and take up painting full time; today I make a living doing what I love to do! I fall asleep feeling good about the day's work and I'm excited to jump

> **Redd Flag**
>
> If the immune system has destroyed a patient's thyroid to the extent that it is unable to produce the necessary life-sustaining hormones, the patient may need to take thyroid hormones. Failing to do so could lead to dementia, poor bone growth and other problems.[35] Remember: Never stop any medications without your prescribing physician's approval.

out of bed in the morning. My husband was always there for me, but today we're back to the closeness we shared when we first met in college.

I do still have days when I'm a little low, especially during my menstrual cycle, but it's manageable. I consider this a huge success. Now that I know how to help myself stay well, it's opened up a whole new possibility for my husband and me. We'd talked about having children in the past, but I was so unhealthy that I was terrified at the thought of being pregnant; I knew there were countless problems that could arise for the baby and me if I was unwell. Now that I'm well and know how to keep my immune system in check, the likelihood that I'll be able to conceive and have a healthy baby is sky-high. We're looking forward to starting our family in the next few years.

CHAPTER 13

Leave No Stone Unturned

Emily F.'s Story

Emily has a very active lifestyle as a wife and mom of four kids. Her family regularly enjoys camping and fishing, four-wheeling, and sports. She's active in her community and church, and is on the board at one of her children's schools. At age 43, Emily was having no trouble keeping up with her hectic and busy life. Then, suddenly, her health plummeted.

Emily's story is unique because her health, abundant energy, and fun-filled lifestyle deteriorated so quickly. Many low thyroid and Hashimoto's patients struggle for years or even decades with worsening symptoms. Emily's health crashed practically overnight.

◇◇◇◇◇◇◇◇◇◇◇◇◇◇◇◇◇◇◇◇◇◇◇◇◇◇◇◇

"I wish I could find the words to describe what a complete turnaround I experienced with my health. When I started my care plan, I was going to bed around 3 p.m. every day; my body just couldn't move any more. It was like all of my muscles shut down, and just lifting an arm or a leg was impossible. Within six weeks of starting my care plan I was awake and active until 9 p.m."

◇◇◇◇◇◇◇◇◇◇◇◇◇◇◇◇◇◇◇◇◇◇◇◇◇◇◇◇

My health problems reached a crisis point in late 2012 when I had surgery for a melanoma. I hadn't been feeling great for about a year at that point, but it was nothing I could really put my finger on. I've always thrived on and preferred a fast-paced lifestyle, and I was doing all the things I always did—going to my kids' sports games, helping out with fundraisers for church and benefits in the community—but I was operating just a little bit slower. It wasn't anything anyone else would necessarily notice, but everything in my life was slowing down.

The surgery marked the beginning of an unhappy, painful, and frightening time for me. I had surgery on my leg, and my life came to a complete standstill for an entire week. This was the first time I'd ever been basically confined to home, and I really couldn't do much at all to take care of myself.

Unfortunately, I didn't recover; my leg just wouldn't heal. After weeks and weeks without improvement, I was finally diagnosed with Hashimoto's disease. It didn't change the course of my care or the decline in my health, but at least I had some clue why I hadn't been feeling well for the past year, and why I couldn't just get over this surgery and feel better.

The day after Christmas, I had my first visit to an urgent care facility. I was so exhausted that I couldn't stay out of bed for longer than two or three hours at a time—I was so lacking in strength and energy that I literally could not hold up my head. I couldn't go outdoors because I was so chilled. I just couldn't get warm, and I had to climb into a hot bath to try to stop shaking.

Redd Flag

This is a good example of how each person suffering with low thyroid can have drastically different symptoms depending on the underlying cause of their condition.[36] If the primary cause of a patient's hypothyroidism is an autoimmune disease, inflammation can occur throughout the entire body. The autoimmune disease can also create many different symptoms because 25% of individuals with one autoimmune disease develop other autoimmune diseases that impact various body systems.[37] When multiple body tissues are under attack from various autoimmune responses, the patient will experience symptoms specific to each autoimmune disease.

Within five days of that first visit, I was back at the ER. Five days after that, I had to go to the ER again. No matter what the medical professionals tried, I kept getting sicker and sicker. Nobody could pinpoint what was wrong.

The problems I had were unlike anything I'd ever experienced. I had severe intestinal problems: pain and uncontrollable diarrhea. My entire body felt achy, especially my joints. I was so uncomfortable I couldn't sleep. I was weak and dehydrated, and suffered from exhaustion and severe headaches. My leg still wasn't healing, so I had pain and swelling from that, too.

The urgent care and hospital staff gave me fluids, pain pills, advised me to get plenty of rest, and put me on antibiotics—nothing helped. I'd been diagnosed with Hashimoto's disease, but nobody seemed to know what to do about it.

Finally, I was referred to an endocrinologist who put me on thyroid medication. It was a "normal dose," and I was told it typically takes about six weeks for the medicine to work. He said I probably wouldn't even notice any effects from taking it.

Within 12 hours of taking the hormone, I had a horrific and terrifying reaction: I became extremely sick; my heart was racing; I had extreme diarrhea, and my blood pressure was sky high. Basically, everything that could go wrong did go wrong. I called my endocrinologist and he insisted it couldn't possibly be a reaction to the medication. He said there was no way I could be reacting to the drug in less than 24 hours. He told me I needed to keep taking it, so I did.

The second day, I had an even stronger reaction. I became more and more dehydrated, and I could feel my heart pounding in my chest. I called my endocrinologist again and told him I'd need to go back to the ER if he didn't do something. He took me off the medication. Within twelve or so hours, I felt better. But I was still sick.

We tried different doses of different medications for three weeks, and I ended up in the ER again. My thyroid levels were all over the place, bouncing up and down according to whether or not I took medication. It was an extremely stressful and frightening time—I had never been more than slightly sick a day in my life!

Eventually, my practitioner prescribed a dose of thyroid medication and told me to take it for an entire week *no matter what.* The goal was to see what would happen. By the end of the week, I'd lost 15 pounds and was so sick I ended up back in the ER. This time, my heart rate was so irregular that I had to see a cardiologist. I also had to see a gastroenterologist because my digestive system was a disaster, and I started seeing a wound specialist because my leg wouldn't heal. My body was in crisis.

Things quickly went from bad to worse. My experience isn't at all common—either in its severity or in how swiftly my health declined. I believe I was already suffering thyroid-related problems, but at a low enough grade that they weren't too troublesome. My body was just too fatigued to recover from surgery. I crashed.

The bright side was a fourth referral from one of the ER doctors to an internal medicine doctor he thought could help me. It turned out to be a great referral. The new practitioner put me on the lowest possible dose of thyroid medication—a dose lower than he'd ever seen anyone put on. Picture the smallest pill you can imagine, and then cut it into quarters. Most people would say, "Don't even bother taking that tiny amount." But it made a difference for me then, and still does today.

What this internal medicine doctor noticed was that, for whatever reason, my body is highly sensitive. He advised me to get on a really good health program, and he would balance my medication. He recommended that I work with someone who could help me learn how to eat properly for my condition. He told me he didn't know enough about that field to be able to help me, so it became my job to find someone who could help me help myself through food.

I wanted so badly to feel better. I went online and searched for every practice I could find that worked on healing the body through food. I asked friends, family, and everyone I talked to for help finding what I needed.

Until that point, I'd been scared to death. After all the sickness and urgent care and hospital visits, who wouldn't be? I was afraid I wouldn't be able to carry on—to live life as I always had. The good health I'd always enjoyed had disappeared, and I was going backwards instead of forwards, getting worse instead of better. I never did stop trying to help myself, and in February of 2013, it finally paid off.

About three weeks after I met with my internal medicine doctor, I found exactly what I was looking for. Within one week, two different people recommended the same healthcare provider. His practice focused on managing thyroid conditions and Hashimoto's disease with a natural, nutrition-based approach.

I was incredibly fortunate to find this practice, and I now realize just how lucky I am that I had a medical professional encourage me to seek this kind of help.

At my first consultation at the new practice, the health advisors and I learned about each other. They asked a lot of questions about my condition and how I was feeling. When I explained how sensitive my body is, I felt like they really listened. Then, they explained how they work and what they offered: an individualized, evidence-based approach using nutrition and supplementation to address my imbalances. They would test my digestive tract, adrenal glands,

Redd Flag

When practitioners are able to work together for the benefit of a mutual patient, the sky is the limit. Emily's internal medicine doctor was great to work with. He knew there was a lot more to her thyroid problem than just the need for thyroid hormone medication, and he was willing to refer her out. Working in conjunction with Emily's doctor made all the difference in her care.

and food sensitivities. These were exactly the same tests my internal medicine doctor had said he'd like me to have done, and I felt confident

I was finally on the right track. These practitioners were eager to work hand in hand with my internal medicine doctor, and it was great to see these brilliant minds come together to benefit my health.

I started the food-based plan and continued seeing my internal medicine doctor. I couldn't have hoped for a better experience. My new practitioner and internal medicine practitioner worked together, so all my providers saw my lab results and knew exactly what was going on. My health was carefully monitored from the moment I started the anti-inflammatory diet and supplements with the new practice, and my sensitivities were taken into careful consideration.

Working together, we decided it would be best for me to go through my care plan at a slow and careful pace—it would take me an entire year to complete my care plan. Where other people may be able to have new foods introduced into their diet every few weeks, my body just couldn't handle it. If I have any reaction at all to a food, it takes me weeks to get back to normal. This happened not long ago with soy. After trying a very small amount of soy, my entire body swelled and the bottoms of my feet became covered in blisters. It took two weeks for me to recover. So, we are taking things very slowly. I'm very patient and so are my healthcare providers.

I've heard other patients at the practice say they've seen results within just a few days or a week of changing their diet and adding supplements. For me, it took a little longer, but my progress was still remarkable.

When I first started my care plan, I had a travel date coming up within four weeks. I was in crisis mode at that point; I literally could not leave my house or stay out of bed for more than a few hours, but I really needed to travel. I asked my new practitioners if they believed it was possible for me to get healthy enough to travel and they said, "We'll find out!"

I avoided the foods I was intolerant to and took the supplements they gave me. Sure enough, I was on that plane on schedule, and I did fine. I was by no means back to "normal," but I could function. I needed time to recover when I returned home, but just the fact that I could do something like that at all was amazing!

I began my care plan in February. By April, I was functioning at about 80% of where I had when I was healthy. I asked them if they thought I'd ever be able to live life the way I used to, and they said they believed it was possible.

Sure enough, by June, I was almost there! My energy levels and "good days" were still improving. Over the summer, I began feeling like my healthy self about 20 or so days out of the month. I realized that if I pushed too hard, I really hurt my body's ability to function. I still have some bad days, but most of the time my body's functioning the way it should!

I wish I could find the words to describe what a complete turnaround I experienced with my health. When I started my care plan, I was going to bed around 3 p.m. every day; my body just couldn't move any more. It was like all of my muscles shut down, and just lifting an arm or a leg was impossible.

Within six weeks of starting my care plan I was awake and active until 9 p.m. I was exhausted by that time, and would sleep like a rock for the whole night, but it was a massive improvement! By the end of the summer, I could stay up if I needed to. If one of my kids needed a ride at 11:30 p.m., I could do it; I could stay up and wait for my daughter to come home from dates. I couldn't stay up late every night, but I was thrilled that I could do it at all.

Although I'm back to my old normal self about 20-25 days a month, I do still have some bad days. I know right away when I wake up if I'm going to have a bad day, and I've learned to give in to not being well. Trying to push through it is the worst thing I can do. I need that day to recover, so I cancel any plans I may have had and just take it easy. I've learned how to manage my own health. Sometimes I don't feel well because of something I ate, and I can pinpoint that and avoid it in the future. Other times, I'm just not well. It's part of living with and managing Hashimoto's disease.

As it turns out, food was the most crucial part of my healing. It requires a lot of patience to go through foods individually and systematically to learn how you react to them. I've learned so much about my body and how it works, and I can quickly tell if I have any inflammation or if I have a flare up or reaction. One of the things I love the most is that my new practitioner doesn't just tell me what to do—he educates me about why we're doing what we're doing. This way I know how to prevent flare ups, and what to do if it happens again.

Although this program was primarily food and supplement based, there was so much more to it. I quickly understood why my internal medicine doctor said he lacked the expertise to help me himself. There is so much to watch out for, monitor, and adjust throughout this program. On top of that, everyone's body is different, so each person has to have an individualized course of care and level of support.

As an example, I had a reaction to some supplements I was taking three days after starting them. I got my practitioner's team on the phone immediately, and explained what was happening. They helped me figure out why the supplement was irritating my body, and quickly recommended another product that would work for me.

This isn't just a "one size fits all" approach, or something someone could do at home on their own. It was completely customized for me. I have a sister who has Grave's disease, and she's now under the care of my health practitioner. It's been fascinating and fun for us to see how different we are—some things that work for her did not work for me. Our care plans are very different even though we're sisters!

One thing my sister and I have both experienced is a kind of realization and acceptance. When you start feeling better after being so sick, you're naturally very grateful to have found something that works—help that makes you feel better. But then you realize that this thing that works requires commitment; it's an entire lifestyle change for most people.

I can see how my diet and the changes I've had to make have helped my entire family. They don't all eat exactly like me but we have much healthier foods in the house. We're all much more aware of what good nutrition means, and how it looks and feels.

My oldest son is 21 now, and prior to November of 2012 he'd never seen me in bed sick. Not even once. This entire experience was frightening for me, but it was scary for my family, too—especially my husband. My kids didn't really realize how sick I was because they were busy with their own lives and I tried not to overwhelm them with my problems, but my husband knew. He did his best to hide it, but he worried all the time.

Today, everyone is happy I'm my normal, energetic self nearly all the time. Having a family to support me and accommodate my needs has been a huge boost for me, and I'm glad they're aware of how important it is to be healthy.

I have to live as a really healthy and careful eater from now on. That's just how I have to be in order to function. At first I was pretty resentful of that fact—I'd never been on a diet in my entire life—but I wasn't stuck in that angry phase for very long. Instead, I focused on how much better I felt. I settled into my new reality and committed to becoming really good at being a healthy eater. Today, people come to me for advice about food and nutrition!

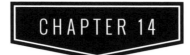

CHAPTER 14

A Natural Approach to Wellness

Emily J.'s Story

A stay-at-home mom of three, Emily was an active, busy person until thyroid problems brought her life to a grinding halt. She had always enjoyed exercise, sports, and the outdoors; then, a year of stress knocked her down to the point where she could barely drag herself off the couch.

Perhaps it was Emily's affinity for nature that led her to seek out natural medicine for what became a major health crisis—or perhaps it was simply a combination of intuition and frustration with the drug-based treatment she had been offered. Whatever it was that drew her to the functional medicine approach that ultimately turned her health around, Emily's story is about trusting your instincts when it comes to your own health. Her story is vitally important for anyone who believes you don't have to accept feeling sick as "normal" when feeling great is an achievable goal.

◇◇◇◇◇◇◇◇◇◇◇◇◇◇◇◇◇◇◇◇◇◇◇◇◇◇◇

"Looking back on this period is hard for me, because everything I used to love and enjoy about life had become a burden too difficult to manage."

◇◇◇◇◇◇◇◇◇◇◇◇◇◇◇◇◇◇◇◇◇◇◇◇◇◇◇

I was in high school when the first sign of hormonal issues surfaced: I had bad acne. I tried every kind of cleanser on the market, and tried watching what I ate. Nothing helped, and the acne persisted. My doctor ordered blood tests, which revealed an adrenal gland issue that was causing my skin problems. The doctor prescribed medication that cleared up my acne, which was a huge relief, but I felt so uncomfortable taking the drug that I stopped the prescription after a while.

Throughout my early 20s, I was healthy and really active. I like to be outdoors, and I enjoy hiking and biking; I love to ski, and I've played tennis since I was in school. I was in pretty good shape when I got pregnant with my first baby. My husband and I were newly married, and we were excited about starting our family. Shortly after the birth of my first child, I started feeling weak. I felt like I was going to faint several times a day.

I went to my family doctor and told him how I was feeling. After running some blood tests and determining I had a thyroid problem, he gave me a prescription. When I asked how long I'd have to stay on it, he said, "Forever." I thought, *No way. You're going to put me on a drug with no explanation and tell me I've got to take it forever?* That just didn't sit well with me.

I went home and shared this information with my mom, who has always been interested in natural healing and holistic health, and she told me my grandmother had also had thyroid problems. My grandmother took thyroid medication all her life, and suffered from its side effects. I didn't want the same thing to happen to me, and I chose not to take the prescription.

> ## Redd Flag
> For nearly 90% of people suffering with low thyroid, the cause is Hashimoto's disease.[9] Our years of experience with Hashimoto's and low thyroid patients supports this statistic—this is what we see in our offices.

Unfortunately, the weakness didn't go away—it got worse. I was confused and I wanted answers. The last thing I wanted was to feel out of control about my own health.

A few months after my regular doctor tried to get me on thyroid medication, I went to see an endocrinologist. After more thorough testing, she diagnosed me with Hashimoto's disease. She said it was a mild case, and explained that when women were pregnant or nursing, their hormones were often all over the place. She suggested I monitor my condition closely during the years I was having children. This diagnosis wasn't much of an answer to how I was feeling, but at least she'd offered me some sort of explanation.

My husband and I planned to have more children after the first, and my thyroid-related symptoms weren't unbearable, so I decided I didn't need to worry about it. Life got pretty busy after our first two babies were born, and the last thing on my mind was regular visits to a doctor. I didn't feel quite right, but I also wouldn't say I was consistently sick.

Unfortunately, life ended up getting pretty stressful. My husband was having a hard time at his job, and we planned to sell our house and make a major move to Arizona. We'd estimated it would take about six months to sell our house, but it ended up selling in four days! We had no place to live and weren't ready to move. We weren't even packed. Right in the middle of this unexpected upheaval, I found out I was pregnant with our third child.

Moving was a big source of stress for me—especially with two small children. We managed to get things sorted, and moved in with my parents until my husband's job could transfer us to Arizona. My daughter was born while we were still living in my parents' home, and she was very colicky. She screamed and screamed for about her first six months, and there was little that seemed to comfort her.

Around this time, I really started feeling like something wasn't quite right with my health. It was December, and although I couldn't quite put my finger on it, something just felt off. I was pregnant again, and I remembered what the doctor had said about Hashimoto's and pregnancy and hormones, so I figured the pregnancy was probably the reason I wasn't feeling right. Things really came to a head shortly thereafter.

I had a miscarriage in March, and began feeling completely exhausted, depressed, and sick to my stomach. Considering all that had happened prior to the pregnancy—an entire year of challenging and stressful events—I didn't think it was odd that I was feeling down. After all, I'd just lost a baby and my husband and I were both struggling emotionally with that. I really thought time and rest would allow me to pull myself back together, but I was never able to do it.

All I wanted was to sit on the couch all day and do nothing. That's all I felt I could physically manage. I didn't want to shop or cook meals or play with my kids because I was too tired. When they were fighting, I didn't have the energy to put up with it. I'd snap at them.

Looking back on this period is hard for me, because everything I used to love and enjoy about life had become a burden too difficult to manage. I'd exercised every day in some form or another for as long as I could remember, but even exercising had become a huge chore. I wanted so badly to be a good mom and partner for my husband—to be in shape and to feel good again. I forced myself to go biking. I tried to keep up with friends who I'd always enjoyed being active with, but I just couldn't do it.

It was difficult to find the motivation to continue doing the activities I had always loved so much. To my husband's dismay, this included intimacy. I'd put my kids to bed at 8:00 p.m., watch TV for half an hour or so, and go straight to bed. I was too tired to stay up or do anything else. I was exhausted. I just didn't have it in me.

It's amazing to me the excuses I came up with for how lousy I felt, and how willing I was to accept that this was somehow "normal." I blamed the exhaustion on having three little kids and trying to do too much. I knew I wasn't thinking clearly. My head felt like it was in a fog all the time. I blamed that on having to run kids around everywhere, and on just being so busy, but not being able to remember basic things just wasn't normal! And, it certainly wasn't normal for me to have zero sex drive.

I wasn't much fun to be around. As bad as I felt, I knew I was also making my husband and kids miserable most of the time. I couldn't handle any amount of stress. I started getting migraines. I was overly emotional. Again, I blamed all this on the stressful year and the miscarriage. Looking at my health realistically, though, I knew there had to be more to it. Time had passed; that year of stress was over.

Finally, in mid-April, my mom suggested I go back and have my thyroid checked again. She saw how my health was affecting me, and she helped me realize that I wasn't going to just snap out of this on my own. I thought maybe she was right. Two people she worked with had thyroid problems, and she asked them for referrals. At that point, I was so sick of feeling lousy and miserable that I decided to look into their recommendations.

The first referral was to an endocrinologist, and the second was to a chiropractic physician who focused on functional medicine and endocrine disorders. I'd already had some experience with a regular endocrinologist, and I preferred the idea of taking a more natural approach to health and wellness. I knew enough to know a chiropractic physician wouldn't just hand me a pill to take and send me on my way. I decided to start with this second recommendation, and made an appointment for a consultation.

In a way, this first visit was like the old saying, "Be careful what you wish for." The practitioner I met with told me there wasn't going to be a quick fix for my situation—you couldn't just put a Band-Aid on poor health. He explained that the type of care his office offered involved looking at the big picture to find the root cause of my health problems. I learned that it would take time, effort, and money for me to return to good health, but that it was possible. Hearing this was a huge relief. For the first time in ages, I had hope of regaining my strength and energy.

I decided to take the necessary steps to start working with the chiropractor, but my husband was a little skeptical about my decision. I can understand why. He's more comfortable with a more conventional approach to health, and he wasn't completely comfortable spending money on "just diets and supplements." Ultimately, he agreed with me because he knew better than anyone how much I had changed and how badly I wanted to be healthy.

The health practitioner ordered extensive blood work, which showed that I was indeed quite sick. I had a whole slew of problems to address: Hashimoto's, hypoglycemia, adrenal fatigue, H. pylori infection, and hormonal imbalance. He created a care plan designed to systematically address these conditions, and set a goal to improve my health within a few months.

I started my care plan with the resolve that I was going to prove to my husband that this natural approach would work. His skepticism actually fueled my determination to feel better and succeed—it turned out to be a good thing! I thank my husband for helping keep me motivated when it sometimes felt like it would be so easy to just give in.

I followed my practitioner's instructions, taking various supplements and modifying my diet, and my symptoms started to improve. It wasn't always easy to stick to the dietary restrictions that my doctor gave me, but I did the best I possibly could. It all paid off.

Now, I feel good all the time. If I make sure to get seven to eight hours of sleep a night, eat every two to three hours, minimize stress, and take my supplements, I feel amazing. I don't get tired or feel sluggish. I don't feel like I want to sit on the couch all day and do nothing. Some days, it seems like my kids wear out before I do—before I'm even done playing with them!

Since I've changed the way I'm eating, I feel light when I'm exercising. Physical activity is no longer a chore, and when I'm biking or playing tennis, I feel energetic. My body can do what I want it to do, and it feels great doing it! I have a bounce in my step.

At this point, I feel good the whole time I'm playing with my kids, cleaning the house, and making dinner. I don't feel tired. I'm thinking clearly now and my mood is much more stable. My libido is back, which is wonderful for my marriage. I've lost twelve pounds in three months without counting a single calorie. I'm not on the couch or in bed as soon as the kids go to sleep; instead, I clean the house, work on projects, or just relax and enjoy spending time with my husband.

Before my health problems reached a crisis point, I'd always thought I was a healthy person. I exercised, followed a pretty healthy diet, and I didn't have weight problems. One thing I've learned during this experience is that a lot of what I thought was "normal" and what other people consider "normal" isn't necessarily normal. It's not normal to feel crappy all the time—to be tired, sluggish, have trouble with mood, sleep poorly, and have little or no sex drive. None of that is normal!

So many of my friends have told me they never even knew I was sick. They ask what I had and what my symptoms were. When I tell them that I just didn't feel right and describe what I experienced, almost every single person says, "Oh, I have that, too. I should go get help like you did. That's exactly how I feel!"

The truth is, I never knew I could feel as good as I feel today. Yes, I'm busy—we're all busy with kids and careers and responsibilities—but a healthy person should have the energy and health to live life without feeling bad. I still have some work to do on my health, but my current energy level is like night and day compared to how fatigued I was feeling before.

Another big thing I've noticed is that the "healthy diet" I was eating was okay, but was by no means great. I used to think I was eating plenty of fruits and veggies and greens. I know now that if you include all the healthy foods in your diet your body needs, there's no room for junk food. When you're eating the right amounts of what you should be eating, there's no craving for a handful of candy here or a donut there; you're not hungry for the junk food. Knowing it will make you feel awful, you just don't want it.

I've learned so much about how my body works and how what I eat affects it. It's amazing to me how quickly things have turned around for my health in just three months! My husband told me the other day that he hasn't once regretted my choice to pursue this natural path to health. He's seen such a change in me, and he's happy I did it because it's really given me back my life. Today, I'm confident that I'll be ready for another pregnancy and will be able to welcome a new baby into my life at the end of this process. It's exciting, and is something my husband and I are really looking forward to.

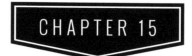

CHAPTER 15

Inspiring Others: You Are Not Alone

Heidi's Story

When Heidi talks about the various challenges she faced as the result of her thyroid problems, her voice is thick with emotion. She was once in a very difficult place physically, mentally, and emotionally, and her memories are powerful. Even though she says, "It isn't fun to go back there," Heidi believes one of the things that helped her the most was hearing other Hashimoto's patients tell their stories. She says she would "hate for someone else to feel as low as she was with nowhere to turn for hope or inspiration." Heidi feels lucky to have had the support of her wife, who encouraged her to seek care. This is her story.

◇◇◇◇◇◇◇◇◇◇◇◇◇◇◇◇◇◇◇◇◇◇◇◇◇◇◇◇◇

"I remember watching online video testimonials of this practice's patients, and everything these people said sounded exactly like me. They had been in my position; they had felt as hopeless, scared and desperate as I did. One day while I was watching these videos, I broke down sobbing. I thought, 'These people picked themselves up and pushed past the fear and got better.' I knew I needed to do the same thing—set aside my fear and do what I needed to do to get healthy."

◇◇◇◇◇◇◇◇◇◇◇◇◇◇◇◇◇◇◇◇◇◇◇◇◇◇◇◇◇

I was in my late thirties when I first found out I had thyroid problems. I had gone to my doctor for just a routine physical and blood work, but my tests showed I had low thyroid. Although I wasn't having any symptoms, my doctor told me I'd have to take thyroid medication and stay on it long term. Naturally, I was alarmed—I felt fine, and my doctor couldn't pinpoint a cause of the low thyroid.

Medication just didn't feel like the right option for me. I don't jump into anything without doing research, and I don't like taking prescription drugs, so I didn't feel comfortable with that course of care. Since there didn't seem to be a cause for my condition and I didn't feel sick, I decided not to take the medication. Instead, I started doing research to find another way to deal with the situation. I'm sure my health declined because of the delay in managing my condition, and it took me two years to finally arrive at what appeared to be an answer: natural medicine.

I found a practitioner I trusted—a naturopathic doctor who I still see today—and he diagnosed me with Hashimoto's disease. He spent a great deal of time educating me about the disease and helping me understand why it was so important for me to address my condition. I felt like my practitioner really understood what was going on with my health, and he explained why he thought I should start taking a natural thyroid hormone replacement. This time, I took the medication.

I hadn't realized just how poorly I'd been feeling until I started to feel a little better. Before taking the thyroid hormone, I had really low energy, aches and pains, and headaches—I constantly felt the way it feels

Redd Flag

If you have a true low thyroid condition, it's crucial to follow the advice of your physician if he or she recommends that you take thyroid hormone. We have seen many patients who don't want to take thyroid hormones because of their commitment to natural medicine. These patients want to find natural solutions to "cure" their low thyroid condition. In my opinion and experience, this is an unrealistic goal.

Research shows that there aren't significant side effects of taking correctly prescribed thyroid hormone. In fact, the benefits far outweigh any risk involved.[38]

when you're about to get a cold or the flu. After taking the hormone replacement, I noticed I could think more clearly and remember dates and names more easily. Although this improved thinking was still far from ideal in terms of mental clarity and physical health, I welcomed the changes.

After a few weeks, my symptoms stopped improving and I began to feel like I was slowly moving backwards. I talked a bit with my naturopathic doctor to try to find an answer, but realized I'd gone as far as I could with his care at that point.

I struggled. It was hard to just make it through the day at work, which was hectic and stressful, and there was nothing I wanted more than to just go home and collapse on the couch and not move. Even though I had initially felt better on my medication, I wanted to do something more; I wanted to go after the root cause of my problems. For me, it wasn't just about treating symptoms—I wanted to actually regain my health.

It wasn't long before I found what I was searching for. I saw a commercial on TV for a health and wellness clinic that focused on diet, supplementation, and nutrition, which seemed to fit with my health goals. I liked the sound of that. They took an evidence-based, scientific approach to thyroid and Hashimoto's care. I thought, *This is exactly what I've been looking for.*

> ## Redd Flag
> This scenario is common, and we call it the honeymoon stage. The patient starts taking thyroid hormone and begins to feel better for a few weeks to a couple of months. Then, they revert back to the way they felt before. This is because nothing is being done to address the main mechanism—the root cause—that is triggering the symptoms.

Even though I had been feeling worse and worse for years, I still hesitated to act. My health was in obvious decline, but the physical discomfort—the headaches, body aches, and exhaustion—just wasn't enough to spur me to take action. It's horribly frightening to know that your health is declining without knowing how to help yourself.

I remember watching online video testimonials of this practice's patients, and everything these people said sounded exactly like me. They had been in my position; they had felt as hopeless, scared and desperate as I did. One day while I was watching these videos, I broke down sobbing. I thought, "These people picked themselves up and pushed past the fear and got better." I knew I needed to do the same thing—set aside my fear and do what I needed to do to get healthy.

My wife had always been a tremendous source of support. She knew everything I'd been through over the past few years, and she'd been by my side the entire time. I was researching this practice and watching testimonial videos and having a hard time knowing what to do, and my wife finally said to me, "Why don't you go and try it?" Her words were just what I needed to finally make up my mind. After all, what did I have to lose? Right in front of me was an opportunity that might end up helping me feel better, and nothing should have held me back—especially not fear! I made an appointment.

When I went in to the office I talked about everything I was feeling and asked the healthcare practitioners a ton of questions. They answered every single one. They were patient with me, and they clearly had a deep understanding of what I was going through; they even seemed to understand my apprehensions. At that point I finally decided, "Okay, I'm doing this," so I took a leap of faith and jumped in.

My care plan primarily involved a pretty strict diet and supplements that addressed my specific imbalances. The diet was pretty intense, but that only lasted a couple of weeks. I started feeling better almost right away, and knowing it was really going to work made it a lot easier to keep going.

The changes were subtle in the beginning, but they were definitely there. The first thing I noticed was that I still had some energy when I came home from work. Instead of conking out on the couch until bedtime, I was walking the dog, doing dishes, and tackling other chores around the house. Before starting my care plan, even those simple activities had felt like mountains that were impossible to climb.

I also had fewer headaches and began to feel a little more in control of my body. I'd been dealing with a lot of achiness in my joints, but the pain lessened; now, it's completely gone.

Things have been much better for me since I completed my care plan. I exercise more, and I enjoy walking our dog again. I am still not 100% every day—sometimes I forget to drink enough water or slip a bit with my diet, but I've learned how to get my health back on track and know that making my health a priority really does make a difference. In the past, I had no idea what to do or what changes I needed to make. Now, I know how to stay healthy, and I'm still

> # Redd Flag
>
> Stopping your exercise routine may sound counterintuitive for someone who wants to feel better. If your health condition is severe, however, exercise could make you feel worse. Intense exercise creates free radicals[39] that can flare up autoimmunity,[40] making symptoms worse for one to three days after exercise.
>
> If you experience intensified symptoms after exercising, decrease the intensity of your exercise to the point where you are able to exercise without aggravating your condition. Once your condition is calmed and your body is functioning at a higher level, exercising can again benefit rather than impair your health.

seeing changes that surprise me in wonderful ways.

For several years before starting my care plan, I'd been participating in an annual event called The Spud Man Triathlon. My sister-in-law had always been my team member; she would swim and run, and I'd do the bike leg of the race. For the past few years, I'd gotten on that bike and couldn't wait for the ride to be over—I had no motivation to do it, and I was completely exhausted for days afterwards.

Last summer, after completing my care with the clinic, I found out at the last minute that my teammate wasn't going to be able to do the triathlon. Two weeks before the event I decided I would do the swim as well as the biking, and my brother would do the run. I started training. When I finished with the swim and the bike ride on the day of the race, I said to myself, "Wow, I could keep going. I could do this whole triathlon myself!" I realized my body was so much healthier than it had been in years. It was such an amazing experience.

Before, I'd never had the desire or motivation to race without a teammate; at that point, I felt so good that I wanted to do the entire triathlon. The following year, I completed all three legs of the triathlon by myself, and I was able to finish it feeling strong! I felt so grateful to have my health back, and I plan to compete again this year.

This has truly been an incredible and eye-opening experience. I'm so thankful I found care providers who understand my health, and received the personalized care that works for me. I got my life back, and I know it wouldn't have happened any other way.

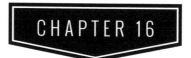

CHAPTER 16

This Is Not the End

If you are suffering from symptoms of low thyroid, I would like to share some tips that may help you take the first steps toward better health. Hopefully, by following some or all of these recommendations, you will begin to feel relief from your symptoms.

1. Identify and remove foods from your diet that exacerbate your symptoms.
2. Make sure your vitamin D levels are within normal range.
3. Drink plenty of water.
4. Avoid simple sugars and artificial sweeteners.
5. Eliminate or limit coffee, soda, and caffeinated beverages.
6. Eat a diet high in vegetables, lean sources of protein, and fruit.
7. Eat frequently throughout the day to stabilize blood sugar levels. To reduce insulin surges, I typically recommend eating every 2-3 hours.

These tips should be applied in conjunction with the advice of your primary care provider. By working with your medical practitioner and following the above suggestions, you may find yourself on the road to better health, wellness, and happiness.

If you have the desire to dig deeper and understand the root cause of your symptoms, seeking the help of a functional medicine provider may be the answer. These providers will address the underlying cause(s) of your condition(s) instead of focusing on specific symptoms.

In your search for a functional medicine provider, I suggest you verify that the doctor is able to order and interpret the following tests. These tests are an important diagnostic tool that will allow your practitioner to better understand and address the true cause of your low thyroid symptoms.

Thyroglobulin Antibody
TPO Antibody
Triiodothyronine (T3)
T3 Uptake
Reverse T3
Free T3
Thyroxine (T4)
Free T4
TSH

Although these tests are an important starting point, this comprehensive thyroid panel evaluates only a small portion of the physiology that can contribute to thyroid symptoms. Your practitioner may recommend additional testing to more thoroughly evaluate your case.

If you are ready to explore this option but are having a hard time finding a trusted and well-respected functional medicine practitioner in your community, call us at RedRiver Health and Wellness Center. We offer support and guidance to patients across the nation and all over the world. No matter which state or country you call home, we are happy to help you navigate the path to better health.

At RedRiver Health and Wellness Center, our primary goal is to introduce our patients to tools that empower them to better manage their own health. When you become a RedRiver patient, you will learn extensively about your own thyroid condition. You will learn what is normal and abnormal for you, and how to prevent or minimize symptoms.

The RedRiver team of healthcare practitioners customizes each patient's care plan to help him or her achieve improved health. With better health comes the opportunity to live a fuller and happier life. We want that for you.

If this book has offered you hope, then my primary objective has been fulfilled. Whether you seek help from RedRiver Health and Wellness Center or from another experienced functional medicine provider, I wish you success on your personal journey to improved health. May courage, hope, and inspiration always be there to guide you. All the best!

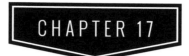

CHAPTER 17

Answers to Common Questions

Some of the most common questions we hear from new patients are, "Are you a doctor? You're a chiropractor, right, so how are you going to help my thyroid problems? Are you going to crack my back to help my thyroid? Can you prescribe my medication? Do I have to take a bunch of supplements? Can you help my child? Can you help me if I don't live in your state?" If you have these questions yourself, you're certainly not alone, and I'm happy to shed some light on these important details.

Chiropractic Physician Education

First—Yes, I'm a chiropractic physician and, as of this publishing, all RedRiver Health and Wellness Center practitioners are chiropractic physicians. I've compiled some data to help you understand a bit more about chiropractic school and the qualifications of chiropractic physicians:

1. The average minimum required classroom hours for graduation from chiropractic school is 2419, and the average minimum required classroom hours for graduation from medical school is 2047.[41] Upon graduation, chiropractic students will have completed an average of 4822 total hours, and medical students will have completed an average of 4667 total hours.[42,43] Both chiropractic and medical students undergo extensive education and training.

2. Chiropractic students often graduate with more training in anatomy, physiology, diagnosis, and the musculoskeletal system than the average medical student.[42,44]

3. The chiropractic curriculum includes anatomy with human dissection, physiology, pathology, microbiology, public health, biochemistry, differential diagnosis, radiology, and various therapeutic techniques.[43]

4. Chiropractic physicians are categorized as primary care providers.[45]

5. While medical schools typically offer few or no core classes in nutrition, chiropractic schools usually offer at least two core courses in nutrition.[46]

6. Like medical doctors, chiropractors are subject to licensing and overview by national and state boards. Chiropractors are required to pass a four-part national board exam in addition to the required state board exams.[41]

While it is clear that chiropractic physicians receive a thorough and diverse education, there exists much room for improvement in the area of nutrition curriculum for both chiropractic and medical schools. Personally, I chose to attend Parker University's chiropractic program because it was one of the top schools—traditional medical or chiropractic—for nutrition and neurology.

The truth is, medical and chiropractic school education is not enough. Over the years, I have acquired a Master of Science in Human Nutrition and Functional Medicine, countless certifications, and two diplomates— one in functional medicine and one in integrative medicine—and have benefitted from the close mentorship of Dr. Datis Kharrazian, who is well known for his work with autoimmune, chronic, and neurological disorders.

As a practitioner who uses dietary, nutraceutical, and lifestyle modification to address complex endocrine and autoimmune conditions, it is critical that I have sufficient education and experience to address the needs of our patients. I am continually furthering my education and expanding my knowledge. It is also important that my colleagues at RedRiver Health and Wellness Center share my passion for outcome-based care and are highly educated and trained. For this reason, I personally mentor each and every practitioner who joins my practice so that we are able to work as a cohesive team of informed, proactive practitioners.

Functional Medicine

So, what is functional medicine? Excellent question. Functional medicine is focused on identifying and addressing the root cause of disease to help patients achieve and maintain optimal wellness. Functional medicine practitioners, like myself and other RedRiver chiropractic physicians, seek to understand each patient's unique story—we recognize that an individual's lifestyle factors and environmental exposures are just as important as genetic factors for the management of chronic disease. In contrast, traditional medicine is focused on identifying and treating isolated symptoms of disease, often ignoring the myriad factors that contribute to the development of the disease itself.

Functional medicine providers practice in all fields of medicine. Although we at RedRiver do address musculoskeletal concerns through chiropractic manipulation, our practice focus is on autoimmune, thyroid, and other endocrine disorders, and we address these conditions using functional medicine techniques. My Diplomate in Functional Medicine required 300 hours of postgraduate work and a functional medicine board examination. I use this training in combination with my Doctor of Chiropractic, MS in Human Nutrition and Functional Medicine, various certifications, and valuable experience each and every day with my patients.

Prescription Rights

Although chiropractic physicians in the United States are qualified to diagnose and manage disease, we do not have DEA numbers to write prescription medications. At RedRiver Health and Wellness Center, we work closely with our patients' prescribing primary care physicians and specialists to provide comprehensive, individualized care.

Nutraceutials

While we at RedRiver don't often rely on prescription drugs to address our patients' various health concerns, we do use several effective tools to help improve the physiological imbalances that cause undesirable symptoms. Nutraceuticals are one such tool.

The physician who coined the term nutraceutical defines it as a food or derivative of food that provides health benefits. Vitamins, minerals, herbs, food, fish oils, and food-based products such as extracts and antioxidants fall into the category of nutraceuticals when they are used to address health-related problems.[47]

When prescribed correctly, nutraceuticals can significantly improve a patient's health. At RedRiver Health and Wellness Center, we don't believe that patients should take handfuls of supplements for the rest of their lives. Instead, we use corrective supplementation in combination with dietary and lifestyle changes to address specific imbalances. Once each physiological imbalance has improved and the supplement is discontinued, the patient is often able to maintain this renewed health simply by continuing his or her recommended diet and lifestyle changes.

Every patient is different, and every patient requires individualized care to address his or her specific needs. There is no single nutraceutical formula that leads to improved health for everybody; among ten Hashimoto's or ten low thyroid patients, each one will require unique dietary modifications, targeted supplementation, and personalized lifestyle modifications. For this reason, it is critical that healthcare providers run the diagnostic tests necessary to determine the underlying cause of each patient's condition. Only then can we recommend the appropriate nutraceuticals to address specific imbalances.

Pediatric Care

It is not unusual for a RedRiver patient to ask if we can provide care for his or her child or teen who is experiencing unexplained symptoms. Our response is, "Yes—autoimmune disease does not discriminate." Children do indeed suffer from autoimmune disorders such as juvenile arthritis, lupus, and celiac disease. Because autoimmunity can run in families, a patient with autoimmune disease may have children with autoimmune disease.[48]

Helping children can be an incredibly rewarding experience for healthcare practitioners. Imagine what would have happened if your health condition had been identified and addressed when you were a child—instead of suffering for years with symptoms of an undiagnosed condition, you would have received the invaluable gift of wellness much earlier in life. Since autoimmune diseases are often progressive, catching them in children and teens can result in a significantly improved quality of life. We welcome the opportunity to help improve the health of children.

Telemedicine

Patients contact RedRiver Health and Wellness from all over the world in the hopes that we can help them find relief from their autoimmune, thyroid, and other endocrine conditions. Many are surprised to learn that RedRiver practitioners are happy to work with them via videoconferencing or telephone, and that our techniques are just as effective from afar. By coordinating testing and care with our patients' prescribing physicians, we are able to help a patient in Dubai just as easily as we can help a patient in our very own community.

◇◇◇◇◇◇◇◇◇◇◇◇◇◇◇◇◇◇◇◇◇◇◇◇◇◇◇◇◇

Hopefully, I've answered some of your questions. If you find yourself wanting to know more about RedRiver Health and Wellness Center, if you have questions that remain unanswered, or if you are interested in scheduling a consultation with a RedRiver practitioner, please visit www.RedRiverHealthAndWellness.com. We are here to help.

About the Author

Joshua J. Redd, DC, MS, DABFM, DAAIM, a chiropractic physician, is the owner and founder of RedRiver Health and Wellness Center. He is highly trained and experienced in managing the care of patients with thyroid disorders, Hashimoto's disease, and other autoimmune conditions. To identify and address the root cause of his patients' challenging immune, endocrine, and neurological disorders, Dr. Redd uses evidence-based functional medicine techniques that allow him to help his patients achieve and maintain optimal health. By working in conjunction with his patients' primary care physicians and endocrinologists, Dr. Redd is able to help domestic and international patients alike who come to RedRiver Health and Wellness Center seeking help and guidance.

Dr. Redd has a BS in Health and Wellness, a BS in Anatomy, and a MS in Human Nutrition and Functional Medicine. He earned his Doctor of Chiropractic from Parker University.

Additionally, he has certifications in the following areas: Mastering Functional Blood Chemistry, Functional Blood Chemistry Analysis, Mastering the Thyroid, and Mastering Brain Chemistry. He has also received certifications from the American Board of Functional Medicine in the following areas: Functional Immunology, Functional Gastroenterology and Functional Medicine.

Dr. Redd has a Diplomate in Functional Medicine from the American Board of Functional Medicine, and a certification and Diplomate in Integrative Medicine from the American Association of Integrative Medicine.

In 2010, Dr. Redd was responsible for hiring the medical staff for the Utah Blaze arena football team, and in 2012 he was selected to be on a panel of doctors for the First Lady of Utah's Conference. He is a board member for the B-Strong Foundation and is also a health consultant for ABC4.

Dr. Redd often co-hosts ABC's *The Younger You*, and his episodes on colon health and brain health were nominated for Emmys. He is also cited in Dr. Datis Kharrazian's book, *Why Isn't My Brain Working?: A Revolutionary Understanding of Brain Decline and Effective Strategies to Recover Your Brain's Health.*

Dr. Redd has spoken at many venues across the nation, teaching patients how to better manage their conditions with nutrition, diet, and lifestyle modifications. He travels across the country lecturing on the following topics: the neuroendocrine immunology of exercise, small intestinal bacterial overgrowth, gluten sensitivity and celiac disease, the gluten/leaky gut/autoimmune connection, functional blood chemistry, and mastering the thyroid.

Since 2010, Dr. Redd has been teaching a weekly religious studies group at the state prison in the women's section. He devotes a large part of his life to service in the community and his church.

"Helping patients regain their health is one of the most gratifying parts of my life. One of my primary goals is to educate patients about their individual conditions and provide them with the tools they need to stay healthy."
— Dr. Joshua Redd

Connect with RedRiver Health and Wellness

RedRiver Online

Website
www.RedRiverHealthAndWellness.com

Facebook
www.Facebook.com/RedRiverHealthAndWellness

Twitter
@AskRedRiver
www.Twitter.com/AskRedRiver

Pinterest
@RedRiverRecipes
www.Pinterest.com/RedRiverRecipes

Instagram
@RedRiverHealthAndWellness
www.Instagram.com/RedRiverHealthAndWellness

Endnotes

[1] Womenshealth.gov. Hashimoto's disease fact sheet. http://womenshealth.gov/publications/our-publications/fact-sheet/hashimoto-disease.html. Updated July 16, 2012. Accessed January 5, 2015.

[2] Amino N. Autoimmunity and hypothyroidism. *Baillieres Clin Endocrinol Metab.* 1988;2(3):591-617.

[3] Veronelli A, Mauri C, Zecchini B, et al. Sexual dysfunction is frequent in premenopausal women with diabetes, obesity, and hypothyroidism, and correlates with markers of increased cardiovascular risk. A preliminary report. *J Sex Med.* 2009;6(6):1561-8.

[4] American Thyroid Association. Hypothyroidism. Thyroid.org website. http://www.thyroid.org/what-is-hypothyroidism. Published May 21, 2012. Accessed January 5, 2015.

[5] Ross, D. Patient information: Hypothyroidism. http://www.uptodate.com/contents/hypothyroidism-underactive-thyroid-beyond-the-basics#references. Updated December 5, 2013. Accessed January 5, 2015.

[6] Kharrazian, D. *Why Do I Still Have Thyroid Symptoms? When My Lab Tests Are Normal, A Revolutionary Breakthrough in Understanding Hashimoto's Disease and Hypothyroidism.* Elephant Printing LLC; 2010.

[7] Boelaert K, Newby PR, Simmonds MJ, et al. Prevalence and relative risk of other autoimmune diseases in subjects with autoimmune thyroid disease. *Am J Med.* 2010;123(2):183.e1-9.

[8] Vertesy L, Beck B, Bronstrup M, Ehrlich K, Kurz M, Muller G, Schummer D. (2009, January 27). Cyclipostins, novel hormone-sensitive lipase inhibitors from Streptomyces sp. DSM 13381. II. Isolation, structure elucidation and biological properties. *The Journal of Antibiotics, 55*(5), 480-494.

[9] Holtorf, K. Insulin resistance can trigger Hashimoto's disease. http://www.nahypothyroidism.org/insulin-resistance-can-trigger-hashimotos-disease. Published April 10, 2013. Accessed January 5, 2015.

[10] National Institute of Diabetes and Digestive and Kidney Diseases, National Institutes of Health. Insulin resistance and prediabetes. National Diabetes Information Clearinghouse website. http://diabetes.niddk.nih.gov/dm/pubs/insulinresistance. Published June, 2014. Updated September 10, 2014. Accessed January 5. 2015.

[11] Puchalski CM. The role of spirituality in health care. Proc (*Bayl Univ Med Cent*). 2001;14(4):352-7.

[12] Gerstmann, L. Immune deficiency and autoimmune disease: A complicated relationship. IG Living website. http://www.igliving.com/magazine/articles/IGL_2009-06_AR_Immune-Deficiency-and-Autoimmune-Disease-A-Complicated-Relationship.pdf. Published June/July 2009. Accessed January 5, 2015.

[13] Arrieta MC, Bistritz L, Meddings JB. Alterations in intestinal permeability. *Gut*. 2006;55(10):1512-20.

[14] Kharrazian, D. Top 10 reasons Hashimoto's patients don't get better. Dr. K News website. http://drknews.com/10-reasons-hashimotos-patients-dont-get-better. Published February 5, 2014. Accessed January 5, 2015.

[15] Kitts D, Yuan Y, Joneja J, et al. Adverse reactions to food constituents: allergy, intolerance, and autoimmunity. *Can J Physiol Pharmacol*. 1997;75(4):241-54.

[16] Rose, N. The common thread. American Autoimmune Related Disease Association website. http://www.aarda.org/autoimmune-information/the-common-thread. Accessed January 5, 2015.

[17] Cárdenas-roldán J, Rojas-villarraga A, Anaya JM. How do autoimmune diseases cluster in families? A systematic review and meta-analysis. *BMC Med*. 2013;11(1):73.

[18] Chakraborty P, Goswami SK, Rajani S, et al. Recurrent pregnancy loss in polycystic ovary syndrome: role of hyperhomocysteinemia and insulin resistance. PLoS ONE. 2013;8(5):e64446.

[19] Janssen OE, Mehlmauer N, Hahn S, Offner AH, Gärtner R. High prevalence of autoimmune thyroiditis in patients with polycystic ovary syndrome. Eur J Endocrinol. 2004;150(3):363-9.

[20] University of Arizona. Putting the brakes on inflammation: Signal prevents immune system from spinning out of control. ScienceDaily website. www.sciencedaily.com/releases/2013/07/130723103456.htm. Published July 23, 2013. Accessed January 6, 2015.

[21] Ricciotti E, Fitzgerald GA. Prostaglandins and inflammation. *Arterioscler Thromb Vasc Biol.* 2011;31(5):986-1000.

[22] Stojanovich L, Marisavljevich D. Stress as a trigger of autoimmune disease. *Autoimmun Rev.* 2008;7(3):209-13.

[23] Schmaling KB, Sher TG. *The Psychology of Couples and Illness, Theory, Research, and Practice.* Amer Psychological Assn; 2000.

[24] National Institute of Diabetes and Digestive and Kidney Diseases, National Institutes of Health. Hashimoto's disease. National Endocrine and Metabolic Diseases Information Service (NEMDIS) website. http://www.endocrine.niddk.nih.gov/pubs/hashimoto/#treatment. Published February, 2014. Updated My 14, 2014. Accessed January 5, 2015.

[25] Mary Ann Liebert, Inc., Publishers. Hashimoto's thyroiditis can affect quality of life even when thyroid gland function is normal. ScienceDaily website. www.sciencedaily.com/releases/2011/02/110225123029.htm. Published February 27, 2011. Accessed January 6, 2015.

[26] Vertesy L, Beck B, Bronstrup M, Ehrlich K, Kurz M, Muller G, Schummer D. (2009, January 27). Cyclipostins, novel hormone-sensitive lipase inhibitors from Streptomyces sp. DSM 13381. II. Isolation, structure elucidation and biological properties. *The Journal of Antibiotics, 55*(5), 480-494.

[27] Saini, S. Chronic urticaria: Clinical manifestations, diagnosis, pathogenesis, and natural history. http://www.uptodate.com/contents/chronic-urticaria-clinical-manifestations-diagnosis-pathogenesis-and-natural-history. Updated January 6, 2015. Accessed January 6, 2015.

[28] Rottem M. Chronic urticaria and autoimmune thyroid disease: is there a link? *Autoimmun Rev.* 2003;2(2):69-72.

[29] Yadav S, Kanwar A, Parsad D, Minz R. Chronic idiopathic urticaria and thyroid autoimmunity: perplexing association. *Indian J Dermatol.* 2013;58(4):325.

[30] Schmidt CW. Questions persist: environmental factors in autoimmune disease. *Environ Health Perspect.* 2011;119(6):A249-53.

[31] Weibel L, Follénius M, Brandenberger G. Biologic rhythms: their changes in night-shift workers. *Presse Med.* 1999;28(5):252-8.

[32] Carnegie Mellon University. How stress influences disease: Study reveals inflammation as the culprit. ScienceDaily website. www.sciencedaily.com/releases/2012/04/120402162546.htm. Published April 2, 2012. Accessed January 6, 2015.

33 Celiac Disease Foundation. Sources of gluten. Celiac Disease Foundation website. http://celiac.org/live-gluten-free/glutenfreediet/sources-of-gluten. Accessed January 5, 2015.

34 Celiac Support Association. Label reading 101. Celiac Support Association website. http://www.csaceliacs.org/label_reading_101.jsp. Accessed January 5, 2015.

35 Boelaert K, Franklyn JA. Thyroid hormone in health and disease. *J Endocrinol.* 2005;187(1):1-15.

36 National Institute of Diabetes and Digestive and Kidney Diseases, National Institutes of Health. Hypothyroidism. National Endocrine and Metabolic Diseases Information Service (NEMDIS) website. http://endocrine.niddk.nih.gov/pubs/hypothyroidism/index.aspx. Published March 13, 2013. Accessed January 4, 2015.

37 Cojocaru M, Cojocaru IM, Silosi I. Multiple autoimmune syndrome. *Maedica (Buchar).* 2010;5(2):132-4.

38 Gerstein, H. Risks associated with treating hypothyroidism. *Can Fam Physician.* Jun 1992; 38: 1467-1468, 1471-1474.

39 Cooper CE, Vollaard NB, Choueiri T, Wilson MT. Exercise, free radicals and oxidative stress. *Biochem Soc Trans.* 2002;30(2):280-5

40 Ahsan H, Ali A, Ali R. Oxygen free radicals and systemic autoimmunity. *Clin Exp Immunol.* 2003;131(3):398-404.

41 The Grisanti Report. Educational requirements for admission to medical and chiropractic college, and for the MD Degree (Doctor of Medicine) and DC degree (Doctor of Chiropractic). Your Medical Detective website. http://www.yourmedicaldetective.com/drgrisanti/mddc.htm. Accessed January 5, 2015.

42 Morter Health Corner. The education of a chiropractor. Morter Health Corner website. http://morterhealthcorner.com/blogs/the-education-of-a-chiropractor. Accessed January 5, 2015.

43 Fontaine KL. Complementary and alternative therapies for nursing practice. Prentice Hall; 2011:182.

44 American Chiropractic Association. Chiropractic education. American Chiropractic Association website. http://www.acatoday.org/level3_css.cfm?T1ID=13&T2ID=61&T3ID=151. Accessed January 4, 2015.

[45] Kremer RG, Duenas R, McGuckin B. Defining primary care and the chiropractic physicians' role in the evolving health care system. *Journal of Chiropractic Medicine.* 2002;1(1):3-8. doi:10.1016/S0899-3467(07)60021-4.

[46] Holtzman D, Burke J. Nutritional counseling in the chiropractic practice: a survey of New York practitioners. *Journal of Chiropractic Medicine.* 2007;6(1):27-31. doi:10.1016/j.jcme.2007.02.008.

[47] El Sohaimy SA. (2012). Functional foods and nutraceuticals-modern approach to food science. *World Applied Sciences Journal* 20(5): 692.

[48] Rothbard, G. Onset of autoimmune disease in children. Autoimmune Mom website. http://www.autoimmunemom.com/kids-life/onset-autoimmune-disease-children.html. Accessed January 5, 2015.

Index